THE BLACKMAIL DIET

THE BLACKMAIL DIET

John Bear, Ph.D.

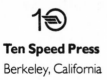

Ten Speed Press
Berkeley, California

Designed by Marc Treib

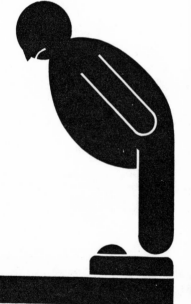

1𝕆

Ten Speed Press
P O Box 7123
Berkeley, California 94707

Library of Congress Catalog Number: 84-50971
ISBN: 0-89815-119-8

10 9 8 7 6 5 4 3 2 1

Printed in the United States of America

TABLE OF CONTENTS

THE SELF-BLACKMAIL PROGRAM

THE WEIGHT-LOSS PROGRAM

REFERENCE

Dedication

Even though all fat people *know* they are fat, sometimes hearing it said by a friend is necessary, because then it somehow becomes more real and unignorable. May everyone be encouraged to worry aloud to their overweight friends — gently or firmly, as the situation requires — that they are, indeed, fat. This book is gratefully dedicated to Lee Carpenter, Mike Young, and Tara Marlowe, the three people who pointed out, advertently or inadvertently, that the Emperor's new clothes didn't fit.

1: INTRODUCTION: WHAT THE BLACKMAIL DIET IS ALL ABOUT

All diet books are useless to the vast majority of their readers, most of whom remain vast.

And I hate them all.

I hate the fact that everybody and his brother who has managed to lose 20 pounds and keep it off for more than three days seems to feel compelled to write a book about the experience.

At least one new diet book is published every week of the year, and they are all, at heart, exactly the same:

1. The author tells how terrible it was to be fat for all those miserable years.

2. He or she describes the major discovery or break-through that finally made weight loss possible.

3. The great discovery is described in detail, along with all the necessary recipes, charts, tables, and procedures.

4. Inspiration, enthusiasm, and encouragement are provided.

I hate all of these books.

I hated them when I was fat, because who wants to read all that terminally smug enthusiasm from some Nouveau Thin neo-celebrity who's probably going to start getting fat again *anyway,* after the last talk-show appearance has ended?

I hate them now that I am no longer fat, because I feel they are, by and large, offering false hope to the needy. Frayed rope to people sinking in quicksand. A map full of misprints when you're lost in the jungle.

Here are three simple and inescapable facts:

1. Of the 80 million overweight people in America today, about 15 million are on a diet of some sort; 65 million are not.

2. Of those who *are* on a diet, about 2 percent will actually weigh *less* in two years than they do now. The other 98 percent may lose some weight, but ultimately they will gain it all back.

3. Therefore, of those 80 million overweight people, less than half of 1 percent will succeed in losing weight.

In other words, out of every 267 fat people in America a grand total of one *is likely to be thinner two years from now than he or she is today.*

What an astonishing failure rate.

What an indictment of an entire industry, when despite all those undoubtedly sincere and well-meaning diet doctors, diet authors, diet counselors, and diet products, the overwhelming majority of the customers fail.

A school that only graduated one out of 267 students would be laughed out of existence at the next meeting of the licensing board.

A pitcher with a one-win, 266-loss record would never make it to the Hall of Fame.

A slot machine that returned one dollar for every $267 poured in would not be permitted, even in the sleaziest Las Vegas dive.

And yet we have Great Diet Discovery after Great Diet Discovery. High carbohydrate from Dr. Solomon. Low carbohydrate from Dr. Atkins. Low protein from Dr. Stillman. High protein from Dr. Tarnower. High fiber from Dr. Reuben. High pineapple from the Beverly Hills Diet. High jinx from Richard Simmons. Like the fat in the gravy, they quickly rise to the top of the bestseller lists.

What's going on here?

Are these authors defrauding or deceiving the public? Most emphatically not, since virtually *any* diet will work, if you stay on it long enough.

Indeed, the most honest and straightforward diet book would contain only these five words: "To lose weight, eat less."

The problem, of course, is that most people don't stay on *any* diet, however good it might be, long enough to lose weight. And of those few who *do* lose weight anyway, 98 percent will gain it back in less than two years.

Diet books can *tell* you what you have to do to lose weight — but they are useless because they cannot *force* you to follow the advice. They can create diets that are supposed to be so easy, so tasty, so much fun, you'll want to stay on them forever. But they cannot *force* you to eat the right food. They can present all the reasons you already know (look better, feel better, live longer, etc.) in new and entertaining and powerful ways. But they cannot *force* you to lose weight.

Rule #1:
The only diet plan that can possibly work, both for losing weight and for keeping it off, is one that somehow does force you to stay on it.

But this is a free country. With few exceptions, people cannot be forced to do things they don't want to do. You will never awake to the sound of a bullhorn: "All right, this is the Diet Squad. We've got the place surrounded. We know you're in there making a triple-dip banana split. Drop your scoops and come out with your hands up." You will never be required to appear for weekly weigh-ins under the watchful eye of the Commissar of Calories. You will never be audited by the Bureau of Internal Residue and forced to explain that package of Oreos you bought at the 7-Eleven last May 17th.

No, the only way you can ever be forced to undertake a major life-changing project is if you bring it upon yourself.

Rule #2:
There are situations in life that you enter voluntarily, but once you have done so, you are no longer in full control of your fate. A successful diet plan must have this voluntary-to-involuntary aspect.

No one is ever forced to get married, but once you *choose* to do so, you come under a whole new set of federal, state, and local laws. No one is ever forced to have a baby, but the moment you *choose* to do so, your life will never be the same. No one is ever forced to buy a house, form a corporation, or sign a contract, but if you *choose* to do so, the process may well be irreversible. In peacetime, people may *voluntarily* join the Army, but having done so, they cannot *voluntarily* leave.

The need, then, is to have a diet plan that you enter voluntarily, but which becomes involuntary and uncancellable once you have begun.

How can any diet plan *force* you to stay with it indefinitely, perhaps permanently?

The answer will come quickly to the minds of all experimental psychologists who may read these words. It is this:

> **Rule #3:**
> **The only kind of diet plan that you would enter into voluntarily, and that you could not easily leave, is one in which the consequences of not losing weight are so unpleasant, you have no real alternative but to lose the weight and keep it off.**

No rat ever *wants* to run through a maze for the sheer joy of running through a maze. The electric shocks it gets for standing still, or turning the wrong way, are a powerful persuasive force. No human ever *wants* to pay his or her income tax. The severe penalties for failing to do so are a powerful persuasive force.

The question to ask, then, is a simple one: what kind of powerful persuasive force would it take to get you to lose weight and keep it off?

Apocryphal and sexist Howard Hughes story:

Hughes (to a woman he's just met): "Would you spend the night with me tonight for a billion dollars in cash?"

Woman: "Why yes, I think I would."

Hughes: "Would you spend the night with me tonight for five cents?"

Woman (indignantly): "What do you think I *am?*"

Hughes: "We've already established that. Now we're negotiating the price."

Let's adapt this to a brief dialogue between you and me.

Author: "Would you enter upon a rigorous diet today, stay on it until you reach your weight-loss goal, and then maintain your ideal weight forever, if I gave you a nickel?"

Reader: "Well, I might *try,* but I couldn't promise . . ."

Author: "Would you enter upon a rigorous diet today, stay on it until you reach your weight-loss goal, and then maintain your ideal weight forever, if I was able to convince you that if you didn't, I'd use my Mafia connections to have your family kidnapped and tortured, your home burned down, and your business destroyed?"

Reader: "Yes, of course I would."

Stephen King has published a splendid little short story, called "Quitters, Inc.," in which the secret of a successful stop-smoking clinic is that the first time a client is seen smoking, they sneak into his house in the middle of the night and cut off his wife's little finger. Of course, there is never a second offense. This story was published several years after the first blackmail diet scheme was implemented. All this proves is that great (or intriguing) ideas can occur to more than one person per decade.

Good. The only question remaining is: What force is powerful enough to get you to start dieting, reach your goal, and stay there?

The answer will be different for every reader.

And that is the topic of this book.

I have no diets to recommend, miracle or otherwise.

I have no handy hints for losing weight through nutrition, exercise, prayer, or any other means.

I have no day-by-day accounts, amusing anecdotes, or inspirational tales of the process by which I lost my 75 pounds.

All I have is a technique that cannot fail. It's as old as the Bible, as modern as the pages of today's newspaper. It is called *blackmail*.

The only "twist" is that you do it to yourself. You willingly enter into an irreversible self-blackmail situation, in which the penalty of failure is so severe, *you literally have no choice but to lose the weight, and keep it off.*

On the next page, I'll describe briefly what *I* did. And then, on the pages that follow, I'll show you how to set up a similar plan for yourself.

Lose weight or else. It's that simple.

What I Did

On Day 1, I put $5,000 into a binding, unbreakable trust. The terms of the trust were as follows: If I lost 75 pounds in the next 365 days, I got all my money back. If I failed to do so, the trustee was to turn the entire sum of money over to the American Nazi Party.

That's all there was to it.

Either I lost the weight or I lost the money.

No compromises. No in-betweens.

And no chance in the world to get out of the deal once the papers had been signed.

Because of the size of the penalty — the importance of that much money to my family and me, not to mention what would happen to the money in Nazi hands — *I literally had no choice.*

So of course I lost the weight.

How am I keeping the weight off? Again, it's very simple. I've signed an agreement with my publisher. If I gain weight, all my royalties from the sale of this book go immediately to the Ku Klux Klan.

I have successfully blackmailed myself.

The same methods can work for everyone.

Whoever you are, whatever your reasons for being overweight, whatever you may have tried before, this method can work. *You can blackmail yourself thin.*

It doesn't require $5,000 — or indeed any money at all.

It doesn't require the cooperation of the American Nazi Party, or any other organization.

There is a self-blackmail scheme for everyone. There are dozens and dozens of different ways to do it. But all the methods have certain principles in common.

In the chapters that follow, I shall discuss and explain these methods and principles, and show you how to set up a blackmail program that can work for you.

In other words, I will teach you how to become a successful — therefore a non-fat — self-blackmailer.

PSYCHOLOGICAL BACKGROUND

Throughout the text, in these sections, I present a little more explanation of the psychological factors at work. Reading them is not essential, but may prove enlightening.

For instance, one thing that makes the self-blackmail scheme work is the fact that many people are willing to *start* something difficult, frightening, or risky, even if they know they won't be able to turn back. I think of this as the Roller Coaster Syndrome. Out of every ten people in a roller coaster car as it reaches the top of the first hill, seven would stop the ride if they could, by the bottom of the first hill. *Knowing* they can't adds to the thrill, of course. Ask any skydiver with one foot out the door of the plane. Ask any person in mid-air, in the process of jumping into an ice-cold swimming pool. Ask any nervous young couple leaving the marriage license bureau.

There is a rush of energy and enthusiasm that gets you over that first hurdle and into the self-blackmail program — even though you know you can never turn back.

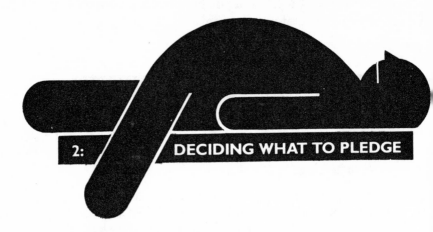

2: DECIDING WHAT TO PLEDGE

The first step in setting up a self-blackmail program is to decide what to pledge. The Pledge is that which you will lose if you fail to meet your weight-loss goal.

It doesn't have to be money. It can be various possessions, your time or talents, or a whole raft of other possibilities, many of which will be discussed throughout this chapter.

First, however, here are some general rules to bear in mind when thinking about what to pledge.

Rule #1:
If you do not reach your weight-loss goal, the penalty must be truly discomforting, crippling, and/or debilitating.

In other words, it's got to hurt. If it doesn't, the temptation may be too great to abandon your horse in mid-stream.

Case History #1:

Pamela G. was 61 pounds overweight. She also used to go bowling two nights a week. (You may have seen her at your local alley. If so, you would not soon forget the sight.) Pamela pledged that if she did not reach her weight-loss goal in six months, she would give up her beloved bowling for one full year.

As time passed, Pamela started thinking that maybe she wouldn't miss bowling all that much, anyway. In fact, the more she thought about it, the more she became convinced of it. And so, by the end of the third month, she had not only dropped out of both her bowling leagues, she had actually started to gain weight due to lack of exercise.

Pamela's self-blackmail failed because the demands of the situation were neither discomforting, crippling, nor debilitating.

Case History #2:

Howard S. was 44 pounds overweight. He was also a stamp collector. And he was an active member of the American Legion. The pride of Howard's stamp collection was an extremely rare zeppelin airmail stamp. Only a few hundred such stamps were known to exist, each one conservatively valued at $5,000.

Determined to lose weight, Howard pledged to donate his treasured stamp to the People's Philatelic Collection of the Moscow State Museum if he failed to reach his goal.

As might be guessed, Howard lost the weight. He reached his goal with six weeks to spare, and the valuable stamp remains safely out of Communist hands.

Rule #2:
If you do not reach your weight-loss goal, the penalty must be realistically enforceable.

There is no point in making a promise if it cannot be kept. If you lose, you *can* pledge to give $1,000 to someone. But you can*not* realistically pledge to "help bring about peace on earth," or to "love your fellow man" (unless, of course, you have a specific fellow man in mind).

Case History #3:

Enid H. was the receptionist for an aluminum tube manufacturer. She had been reprimanded by her employers several times for being snippy, sharp, and sometimes downright rude to visitors, letter carriers, and secretaries, among others. "I thought you fat people were supposed to be jolly," people often said to her.

Enid pledged that if she did not lose the 35 pounds she wished to shed, she would be "nice, smiling, and cheerful to everyone, all the time."

After about three weeks of near-starvation (or so it seemed), Enid decided that it just wasn't worth it. There was no way they could force her to be cheerful anyway, and if they didn't like her the way she was, they could jolly well fire her. Enid is still fat and grumpy. And they fired her.

Rule #3:
If you do not reach your weight-loss goal, the penalty must occur in a reasonably short period of time.

A pledge to give $1,000 on a certain date 25 years in the future is not realistic. Even if you and the recipient are still around in a quarter of a century, by then $1,000 might be the price of a telephone call to Cleveland.

PSYCHOLOGICAL BACKGROUND

It has been well established, both in the psychological laboratory and in the real world, that the longer a punishment comes after the act being punished, the less effect it is likely to have. This is well known by all who have tried to housebreak a puppy. If the puppy "has an accident" on the rug, and is yelled at or swatted at once, it will quickly learn that it did something wrong. If the punishment comes an hour or two after the act, the puppy will have no idea what the punishment is for, and will never learn.

The same phenomenon helps explain why people stay fat or keep on smoking cigarettes. When you remind a heavy 20-year-old smoker that he or she is likely to get lung cancer in 30 or 40 years, the concept of punishment that far away has little effect. If lung cancer struck 21-year-olds in large numbers, their smoking habits would change dramatically.

What's going on here? For most people, the notion of a punishment at some distant time is just not worth worrying about. "I'll cross that bridge when I come to it," they say. When the punishment finally *does* come, like the errant puppy, they may well have no recollection of what they are being punished for.

Thus it is essential that the self-blackmail penalty happen so soon that its mere existence is like a black cloud hovering over you. You know that there will be no time even to *think* about how to weasel out of it.

**Rule #4:
If you do not reach your
weight-loss goal, the
administration of the penalty
must be totally out of your
hands, and out of the hands of
any of your close friends or
relatives.**

You can well imagine situations where a loving spouse
or a devoted friend, entrusted with carrying out the
terms of your self-blackmail contract, simply could not
bring him or herself to deprive you of your money,
possessions, or whatever else you have pledged.

Case History #4:

*Bernard K. was a woodcarver by profession as well as
by hobby. During the day, he worked in the fine-
detailing line at a large furniture factory. In his spare
time, he carved exquisite tiny wooden figures — all the
more remarkable because of his big fat beefy hands.*

*Warned by his doctor about incipient diabetes,
Bernard pledged to lose 48 pounds. His blackmail
plan was that if he did not make his goal, he would be
required to watch while his proudest and most mag-
nificent creation — a complete set of ornate Mediaeval
chessmen, on which he had worked for five years —
would be thrown into the fire.*

*Bernard's big mistake was appointing his wife,
Denise, as trustee. Although Denise was enthusiastic
at the start, after three months, when it became clear
that Bernard simply could not lose weight as fast as he
had pledged, it became equally clear that Denise was
completely incapable of destroying the chess set. "Don't
you worry, Bernie," she said. "You can take a few
extra months if you need them."*

Well, sad to say, after two years, Denise is still extend-
ing the time limit, and while Bernard does lose a few
pounds from time to time, at his present rate of loss he
will be 94 years old before he reaches his goal. He
should live so long.

Rule #5:
Let the penalty fit the
"crime."

The annals of fact and fiction are filled with stories in which a mighty effort is meagerly rewarded. Not long ago, three robbers laboriously dug a half-mile tunnel to get into a bank vault, and once inside found about $50 in cash and a lot of non-negotiable stocks.

There are, on the other hand, situations in which minimal effort is abundantly rewarded, as in the case of the eccentric millionaire who routinely paid for a shoeshine with a $100 bill, saying "Keep the change."

Don't fall into either trap. Don't pledge your entire life's savings, your home, and your first-born son if all you want to do is lose 11 pounds.

On the other hand, a pledge of $50, or giving up golf for a week, isn't going to be much of an incentive to help you lose 62 pounds.

Be realistic. A failure has got to hurt, sure, but don't overdo it.

Don't *under*do it either.

Case History #5:

Lena and Lottie R. were professionally known as "The Tubby Twosome: 555 Pounds of Pure Dynamite." Lottie weighed 289 pounds, Lena a mere 266. When the act broke up, each twin decided to lose 100 pounds.

Lena, whose father-in-law had died in a Nazi concentration camp, pledged to give her entire life's savings, plus 50 percent of her earnings for the next ten years, to the American Nazi Party if she failed.

Lottie, who was a staunch Republican, pledged $100 to the Democratic Party.

Unfortunately, Lena overdid it, and Lottie underdid it.

By the second week, Lena came to realize that if she should fail, not only would she be in truly dire financial straits now, but for many years to come. Her children might not be able to go to college.

Lena tried to get out of the contract, but she found that it was legally ironclad, just the way it should be. Her only alternative was to lose the weight, which she ultimately did, but her level of anxiety rose so high that she had to seek treatment from a clinical psychologist.

On the other, and plumper hand, Lottie's $100 pledge simply did not provide any incentive at all. "I've lost that much in one hour at Las Vegas," she said. "Why should I starve for a year?" She lost almost no weight at all.

Finally, on the advice of a wise friend, she upped the ante to $3,500 and her new Buick station wagon to the Socialist Workers' Party. Then she lost the weight.

Let us review the general rules, and then proceed to the specifics of selecting your pledge:

1. The penalty for failure should be truly discomforting, crippling, or debilitating.
2. The penalty should be realistically enforceable.
3. The penalty should occur quickly.
4. Administration of the penalty should be by an impartial outside source.
5. The penalty should fit the "crime."

The next step in turning you into a successful self-blackmailer is the selection of what to pledge.

PSYCHOLOGICAL BACKGROUND

The question often arises, why not a *reward* instead of *punishment* for achieving a weight-loss goal? There are three good reasons:

1. Many laboratory experiments have demonstrated that punishment is a more effective way of causing behavior change than reward. For instance, in one experiment, two groups of rats were taught to run through a maze. One group received a reward of yummy food when they reached the end. The other group got a nasty electric shock every time they made a wrong turn. The rats in the punishment group learned the required behavior much faster than those in the reward group. Among humans, a typical situation would be the choice between "I'll spank you if you write on the wall one more time," and "I'll give you a candy if you don't write on the wall for one month." Punishment usually works better.

2. It's a lot harder to set up a reward situation. Wouldn't if be nice if some kind-hearted and skinny billionaire would give you $5,000 or $5 million for meeting your weight-loss goal? Most

people would do it under these circumstances. But such a humanitarian has not yet stepped forward. Don't hold your breadth. It is simply far more practical to give away something *you* have, rather than arrange for someone else to give you something *they* have. (The group ante plan, where a bunch of fat people each put up a large sum, the successful losers to divide the spoils, as described on page 00, comes close to this approach.)

3. In a very real sense, becoming thin *is* a reward. And in another very real sense, absence of punishment can be considered a significant reward, in and of itself.

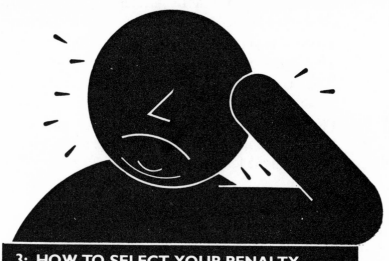

3: HOW TO SELECT YOUR PENALTY

Based on the five general rules presented in Chapter 2, there are seven different categories of pledges — that which you will pay if you don't meet your weight-loss goal. Some are financially painful, some physically painful, some emotionally or psychologically painful, and some have elements of two or all three.

As you read through the following possibilities, examples, and case histories, think about your own personal situation, and how these ideas — or variations on them— might best apply to you.

Category #1: Money, Savings Bonds, or Negotiable Securities

You are the best judge of an amount that will be financially debilitating without being utterly ruinous. I think the absolute minimum should be one month's salary, or one month's total family income.

Other rules of thumb you may wish to consider are:

a. One half (or some other significant fraction) of your total liquid assets.

b. $100 a pound for every pound you want to lose. This is giving your fat roughly the same value as Beluga caviar or pure silver — or 50 times the value of chicken fat.

c. Five percent of your salary for the next year (or two years), on a salary withholding plan, as described in the following section.

Sub-category #1-A:
The Salary Withholding Plan

If you simply do not have the money available now, or if you opt for Rule of Thumb (c), you may consider entering into a salary withholding plan with your employer, if he or she is willing to cooperate.

Your employer would simply withhold a specific amount from each paycheck, and accumulate it for you. Unfortunately, like income tax withholding and Social Security, you would quickly learn not to miss these deductions at all. This is not good. There should be frequent reminders, perhaps with each deduction: "There is now $1,740 in your 'fat fund' — how are you doing?"

If you make your weight-loss goal, then you get a big lump-sum payment, which will seem almost like a cash bonus. And if you don't make it, your employer should make out the check, dangle it in your fat little face, and, with appropriate ceremony, turn it over to the Other Party, whomever.

I think most employers would be willing to go along with this sort of scheme, since (a) it shows your drive, perseverance, and willpower, and (b) it is better for the company, since thinner employees tend to be healthier, more productive, have better attendance records, live longer, and can fit between the aisles in the warehouse.

You may run into a bit of a problem if your *boss* is fat (but maybe you don't want to work there anyway; recent research has shown that a fat boss is likely to be a poor boss).

Of course, if you have good job *and* a fat boss, you could always loan him or her your copy of this book when you're done. Or better still, send a new one. Anonymously, of course.

PSYCHOLOGICAL BACKGROUND

Industrial psychologists obtained a list of America's 100 best-run big corporations, and the 100 worst-run corporations, as selected by a group of experienced stockbrokers and business analysts. Of the 100 best-run companies, *not a single one* had an overweight president! Of the 100 worst-run companies, 32 had an overweight president.

In general, it seems to be the case that a compulsive eater who lacks self-control and behaves irrationally at the dining table is likely to do likewise at the conference table and the bargaining table, to the detriment of his or her company. In fact, some stockbrokers seriously recommend against buying stock in companies with fat presidents.

Category #2: Time, Talent, or Services

The next category of penalties are those involving the pledge of some of your time or talent. But this pledge alone is rarely enough. It should be backed up by a *secondary* pledge of money or other tangible valuables. Otherwise it is just too easy to weasel out of it — and there are laws against involuntary servitude.

Case History #6:

Alex P. was a plumber. A fat plumber. He wanted to lose 37 pounds. So he pledged to do every other job absolutely free for one year if he didn't make his weight-loss goal. He discovered quickly enough that he liked beer more than he liked the idea of being thin. So he failed.

But then, after only four days of doing free jobs, he said, "Nuts to this," and went back to charging his usual $40 an hour, door to door, to all customers. Who (besides his own pudgy conscience) could stop him?

Alex should have backed up his pledge of time or services with a *secondary pledge* of cold hard cash.

Case History #7:

Mary Lou S. was a fervent Southern Baptist. And a fat one. She needed to lose 27 pounds. So she pledged to spend ten hours a week for one year working at the local Catholic Missionary Society headquarters if she didn't make her goal.

Then she made a secondary pledge: *if she failed to spend the full 520 hours during the year helping the Catholic missionaries, then she would pay the sum of $1,000 to the Campaign for Surplus Rosaries. That money was put in a special savings account, with a trustee in charge, so that at least it was drawing interest while the weight-losing program was under way.*

Mary Lou set a time limit of four months, and she was successful in less than three.

Category #3: Valuable Possessions

Valuable possessions must be items that have value for *anyone* on the open market: jewelry, art works, television sets, appliances, cars, golf clubs, and so forth. These are just like money, and should be so treated.

If the objects themselves cannot be given to an independent trustee for safekeeping, as for example with an automobile that you will need to drive, then you should sign an agreement turning title or ownership in the item over to the trustee. A sample form of such an agreement will be found in Appendix D.

Case History #8:

Wanda T. was a middle-aged suburban housewife. Her two favorite pastimes were watching daytime television and eating. As a result, she had a 25-inch color television set and a 38-inch waist.

Wanda's least-favorite person in the entire world was Fannie M., an old busybody who lived a few doors away, and who was forever dropping in, uninvited, to watch television and nibble bon bons. Fannie had a 9-inch black-and-white television and a 22-inch waist.

When Wanda undertook her self-blackmail program, she pledged to give her color television set, free and clear, to Fannie if she didn't meet her goal on time. Wanda and her eagerly cooperating husband Frank (he didn't like television or fat wives) signed an agreement conveying ownership of the television (which cost $749.50, including remote control) over to a lawyer, with instructions to transfer it over to Fannie unless the goal was met.

The prospect of losing her television (Frank made it clear they could not afford another like it) was too much to take. Wanda began doing sit-ups in front of "General Hospital." Although she cut it pretty close, she did reach her goal with a week to spare. Poor Fannie.

Category #4: Treasured Possessions

Treasured possessions are items with no intrinsic or cash value, but which are very important to you. They must not only be important, they must be *totally irreplaceable.*

This category might include, for instance, items like love letters, important photographs, pressed flowers from the high school prom, children's drawings, family heirlooms, and so forth.

The irreplaceability is vital. Otherwise it won't work. I happen to be inordinately fond of a little plastic World War II "British American Ambulance Corps" toy ambulance bank. It cost me 50 cents. I would be quite unhappy if I lost it, but I suspect hundreds of thousands of them were manufactured, so it is inevitable that I would someday find another just like it.

But things like my record album personally autographed by Sharkey Bonnano, or my high school yearbook with its handwritten letter from Margaret O'Brien herself — why, I'd seriously consider losing an extra ten pounds next week to save these from destruction.

Case History #9:

Professor Amos K. has occupied the same office on campus for 22 years. In his office, along with papers and books piled from floor to ceiling, there is a huge brown leather overstuffed chair. The Professor has averaged approximately four hours per day in this chair for 17 years.

When his wife finally badgered him into losing some weight (none of his vests would button up any more), he chose to put up the chair as a pledge. If he failed, it would go forthwith to the city dump.

The problem was that the world is filled with big ugly super-comfortable chairs. Professor K. encountered several at a second-hand store, while ostensibly browsing through used books, and concluded that one of them was perhaps even a bit more comfortable than the one he had been sitting in for 17 years. He had a chocolate eclair for lunch that day, which signified the beginning of the end.

He did not make his goal. True to his word, his old chair went away. Presto, his new one came in. And just like his lectures, nothing at all really changed from that year to the next — including the fact that none of his vests would button.

The big problem in dealing with treasured possessions is to decide (in advance, of course) what to do with them in case you don't meet your weight-loss goal.

What is the worst possible thing that could happen to such artifacts? Most of them you couldn't *give* away. Who, but you, would want them? (Well, how much would *you* pay for a snapshot of Karen Krauskopf standing next to the world's largest helicopter at the Bishop, California, airport in 1958? See.)

I suppose you *could* have things sent anonymously to some remote museum. (The National Peruvian Museum of Trivia at Lima? The Kathmandu Provincial Repository for Worthless Objects?) Or they might be buried in a non-prestigious little time capsule. No, I must reluctantly conclude that the only truly satisfactory disposition of treasured possessions is to have them irrevocably destroyed — preferably right before your very eyes.

Psychologists have determined that people can be divided into three categories: those who are largely *thing*-oriented, those who are *idea*-oriented, and those who are *experience*-oriented. Types are determined by asking questions like these:

1. On a Sunday morning, would you rather (a) go to a flea market, (b) attend a Sunday school class, or (c) watch the sunrise?

2. Would you rather subscribe to (a) *Motor Trend*, (b) *Modern Philosophy*, or (c) *Art Digest?*

3. On a trip to another country, which is most important: (a) taking photographs, (b) meeting the people, or (c) seeing the sights?

In each case, the (a) answer is thing-oriented, the (b) idea-oriented, and the (c) experience-oriented. "Thing" people often find it hard to understand how it is that "idea" and "experience" people can fail to be wired for nostalgia and the joy of possessing objects. Clearly, the treasured possessions option only will work for "thing" people.

Case History #10:

Ronald B. was an impoverished young student. He was plump and had in fact been so since birth (10½ pounds). He suspected that his bulging middle contributed heavily, as it were, to his lack of success with the opposite sex.

Finally, Ronald turned in desperation to self-blackmail. Being very poor, and possessed of few worldly goods, he was at a loss as to what to pledge, and to whom.

After detailed questioning, a counselor was able to determine that Ronald had only one cherished possession: a framed set of Mediaeval music manuscripts. Although their cash value was low, Ronald loved them. And they were truly one of a kind.

Further interrogation revealed that Ronald was essentially non-political in nature, and being a gentle sort, had no particular enemies or hate objects. So the only form of self-blackmail that had any real meaning for him was the threat that his beloved manuscripts would be destroyed as he watched.

An honest and trustworthy roommate was appointed as trustee. If this roommate did not personally observe Ronald standing on the scale in the Men's Gym weighing in at 33 pounds less within five months, he was to remove the manuscripts from the frame, and before Ronald's anguished eyes, tear them into shreds and set them ablaze in the chemistry lab incinerator.

Ronald knew his roommate would carry out the pledge. He was that sort of roommate. During the weight-loss program, Ronald even stooped so low as to visit a few antique and old print shops to see if they had any more manuscripts like his. Fortunately for him they didn't.

And so Ronald lost his 33 pounds with nine days to spare. Twenty-seven days after that he was known to be "going steady" with Mary D., a cheerleader.

Category #5: Second-Party Concessions

This category, and the one that follows, involve actions on the part of a second party, rather than by you yourself. As such, they are less satisfactory, but if nothing else seems relevant — or if there are particular considerations in your own case that give these special appeal — they may well be worth considering.

To utilize second-party concessions, you pledge that someone else, over whom you have some measure of control, will be permitted to do something *they* want to do, but you *don't* want them to do.

Case History #11:

Arthur C. had a 14-year-old daughter who was not allowed to date boys (and dating girls isn't much fun if you are one). Arthur, being somewhat straight-laced, had decreed that Lisa could not date until she was 16. Actually, Arthur's laces weren't all that straight. In fact, they were bulging, since Arthur was 31 pounds overweight.

Arthur pledged that if he did not lose the 31 pounds within 100 days, Lisa would be permitted to date.

Unfortunately, in this case the outcome was clouded, because the 100th day happened to be a Sunday, and Arthur was not weighed officially until his doctor came in on Monday. Arthur claimed he had satisfied the agreement, Lisa claimed he hadn't. Now they've got something new to fight about.

Second-party concessions like this should be put in writing, and although they may not be legally binding, they do have pretty strong moral bonds. Furthermore, they can be backed up by a secondary financial pledge, as in Category #2 above, and in the example that follows.

Case History #12:

Nate S. was an autocratic, almost tyrannical businessman. He was president of a large vegetable cannery, which he had founded many years before. Among his many idiosyncrasies, Nate required all his employees to work half a day on Saturday. "That's the way it was when I broke in, and by gum, that's the way it's going to be now," he often said.

Another of Nate's indiosyncrasies was that he ate four meals a day, five on Sunday, and none of them heavy on his own vegetables. As a result, he had grown heavy on meat and potatoes, almond tortes and egg frappes.

When emphysema nearly prevented him from climbing the stairs to his office — he wasn't about to install one of those newfangled elevators either — Nate reluctantly undertook a self-blackmail program to reduce.

Nate pledged that if he failed to meet his goal, his employees would never have to work on Saturdays again. And, he backed that up with a $10,000 bond, such that if he ever went back on his word, the money would all go to the Draft Resisters' League.

Despite the best efforts of his loyal personnel, who left opened boxes of cookies around the office, signed him up for the Candy-of-the-Month Club, and even tried to spike his coffee with extra sugar, Nate managed to meet his goal. So his employees still work on Saturday — those, that is, who haven't gone to work for the rival firm down the highway. Poor skinny Nate.

There are many other kinds of second-party concessions, most of them falling in the arena of relationships between parent and child, employer and employee, or close friends. They may involve penalties or rewards. For instance, there are such phenomena as underage children who want to get married and need parental permission; use of the family car by teenagers; taking the vacation at the lake (mountains) instead of the mountains (lake); reaching third base, as it were; being transferred to the branch office in Elbow Creek; use (or denial) of a company car; and so forth.

Category #6: Deed Performed (or Not Performed) by a Concerned Second Party

In such situations, a second party who really wants the first party to lose weight (often this is a spouse, significant other, child, or parent) promises to perform (or withhold) certain actions if the first party does not achieve the goal.

There is a good historical precedent here. As Aristophanes recounts the story in *Lysistrata,* the Greek women, desirous that their husbands stop fighting silly wars, banded together and decided to withhold sexual pleasures until peace was restored. I am certain that if the Greek army had been fat instead of belligerent, the same technique would have worked to slim them down, *en masse.*

Similarly, the second party could pledge his or her time to work for an organization despised by The Plump One. For instance, the son or daughter of a staunch Catholic might pledge to work as a volunteer at a local abortion referral center.

It is far better if the would-be weight loser has to suffer directly, but as the Marquis de Sade would say, indirect suffering is better than no suffering at all.

PSYCHOLOGICAL BACKGROUND

The matter of second-hand suffering is one that has interested many psychologists. Kidnappers traditionally play on these second-hand emotions in their ransom notes: do something you really don't want to do (pay lots of money to criminals; donate millions of dollars worth of food to the poor, as Patty Hearst's father did) — or we'll do something you won't like to someone you love.

In a classic and rather unsettling experiment regarding second-hand suffering, Stanley Milgram invited subjects to assist him in what they *thought* was a "learning experiment." The subject was told to keep increasing the size of electric shock being administered to a "victim" each time the victim made a mistake. (The victim was really an actor who was only pretending to suffer, but the subject didn't know that.) In the belief that inflicting this punishment was somehow necessary, 67 percent of subjects continued increasing the size of the shocks they thought they were administering into and beyond a zone clearly labelled "Danger, Severe Shock." Milgram saw this as an alarming case of conformist behavior, and so it is. But it is also a demonstration of the lengths to which second parties will go to assist in what they believe is a valid behavior-changing process.

Category #7: Real Blackmail-Type Blackmail

The final kind of blackmail you might consider is, for want of a better term, Good Old-Fashioned Traditional Everyday Garden Variety Blackmail. (I am indebted to Mr. Jon Ford for pointing out this all-too-obvious option, which had quite eluded me. Mr. Ford purports to be a sales engineer for an envelope company, but with a diabolical mind like his, who can be sure? In any event, it is clear that he has not actually indulged in any of these practices. His somewhat plumpish physique provides, shall we say, ample evidence.)

Consider, then, the nature of classic blackmail — the kind you read about in mystery novels and lurid newspaper stories:

Person A performs Act X. Person A desperately hopes that Person B never finds out about Act X. Person C (the blackmailer) somehow knows about Act X, and tells Person A that he will inform Person B about Act X unless Person A suitably rewards Person C.

But enough abstract discussion. Let's get down to cases.

Case History #13:

Let A = Peter L., a mild-mannered businessman.

Let B = Peter's unbelievably jealous wife, Audrey.

Let Act X = that wild evening at the Housewares Convention last year, when Peter had a glass and a half of champagne, and attempted to kiss a chambermaid in the mop closet. (He succeeded.)

Let C = Peter's co-worker, George B., who, along with Peter, is being considered for the job of Regional Manager.

George let Peter know, one miserable afternoon in the employees' locker room, that unless Peter withdrew from the competition for Regional Manager, George would tell Audrey all about Peter kissing the chambermaid in the mop closet.

And so we have the consequences: in this case, a successful blackmail. Peter felt that given a choice of job or family, he had better choose family. He withdrew, and George became the Regional Manager.

Now that we see how classic blackmail operates, let us replay the above case of deadly white-collar crime, but change it to a weight-losing situation.

Case History #13-A:

The circumstances are identical to the above, except this time Peter L. is fat, and George B. is a sincere friend of his who wants to help him lose weight. This time, Peter decides to blackmail himself.

Peter writes a long letter, telling in excruciating detail about his episode with the chambermaid in the mop closet. He may even get carried away and add a few details that happened only in his fantasies. He seals this letter in an envelope, and gives it to his friend

*George to hold, with the following instructions: "If I
do not lose 35 pounds by August 31 of this year, you
are to mail the letter I have just handed you."*

*Peter's self-blackmail scheme is nearly perfect, and it
did, in fact, succeed. He lost the 35 pounds fully six
weeks ahead of schedule, and the letter was burned
before his very eyes.*

The only potential time bomb in this situation is
Peter's decision to leave the incriminating letter with
his friend George. This may have been unwise.
Incriminating materials should probably not be left
with friends, no matter how close they are. There are
three reasons for this.

One deals with ruptured relationships. What if something happens during the weight-loss period that
destroys the friendship between the two participants?
What if George chose to mail the letter out of spite,
regardless of Peter's performance on the scales?

Another deals with strong friendships. Because he *is* a
good friend, George may well feel sorry for Peter,
and give in to Peter's entreaties that the letter not be
mailed. Could a true friend actually mail a letter which
he knew (or suspected) might break up a happy home?

The third relates to the matter of trusting *anyone* with
anything. What if George dies or becomes ill, and
George's wife Sandra, who never liked Peter that
much, finds and opens the letter? This is why many
people entrust vital documents, objects, etc., not to
friends or *any* individuals, but rather to banks or law
firms. Consider one more example:

Case History #14:

When Kathryn P. was a freshman in college, she was caught cheating on a biology exam, and subsequently asked to leave school. This unhappy event does not appear on her official school records.

A year later, Kathryn enrolled in business school and now, four years later and 43 pounds heavier, she is a bookkeeper for an air taxi service.

The office manager, Kathryn's boss, is scrupulously honest. Overly so, one might say. He has no tolerance for any dishonesty, no matter how slight. Kathryn's predecessor was fired when he learned that her age was actually 41 and not 38, as she had put on her application forms. A clerk was once fired for putting company postage on a personal letter.

Kathryn, desperate to lose weight, wrote a long letter to her boss describing her college indiscretion in great detail. She even went so far as to hint that this was not the only one (although in truth it was).

Kathryn did not have a family lawyer; she gave the letter to her personal physician. It was addressed and stamped, and the physician's instructions were to mail it in five months if she did not come in, get on the scales, and show a 43-pound loss.

As may have been predicted, she succeeded admirably.

By now, many people are saying, "Well, that's all very nice for people with checkered pasts — but what have *I* done that's fair game for blackmail?"

To you clean livers, I can suggest one of the following courses of action:

1. Think harder.
2. Start now. It's never too late.

Let us discuss these two alternatives.

Think Harder

Have you never done *anything* in your entire life that would embarrass or otherwise distress you if it became known to your (a) wife or husband, (b) parents or in-laws, (c) children, (d) friends or co-workers, (e) boss, (f) police department, (g) clergyman, or (h) federal government?

Do you really mean to stand there in your tightly-fitting clothes and say that you never even once fudged on your income tax the tiniest little bit? (If you're so perfect, why did God make you fat?)

Case History #15:

The following self-explanatory letter was written by Thomas W., and left with his lawyer, with instructions to mail it if his weight-loss goal was not reached by a certain date.

Director, Bureau of Internal Revenue
Washington, D.C. 20002

Dear Sir:

My conscience has been troubling me, and I would like to make certain corrections in my federal income tax return for certain previous years. Specifically,

— For the last three years, I deducted $260 each year for religious contributions, representing $5 a week in the collection plate at church every Sunday. Actually, my total church attendance for this period consisted of going to one Easter service two years ago, at which time having forgotten my wallet I put 35 cents in the plate.

— The business trip for which I deducted $672.49 was in fact a pleasure trip, and the "secretary" who accompanied me to Mexico City was in fact my wife.

These are the only discrepancies that come to mind right now, but I'm sure that if you were to look at my returns for other recent years, you might well find additional points to question.

Sincerely yours.

The author of this letter reached his weight-loss goal of 51 pounds with plenty of time to spare, and his lawyer destroyed the incriminating evidence, unopened.

Do Something Now

If you've truly never done anything that is blackmail-worthy before, and you genuinely want to lose weight, it's not too late to start now. Whatever you choose to do must be genuinely felt, and impossible to weasel out of.

For instance, you might write a letter to the well-known politician you dislike the most, telling him or her what you'd *really* like to do *to* or *with* him or her. Be sure to pick one with FBI or Secret Service protection.

Perhaps a similarly candid letter to your boss.

If you felt like it, you could also address an obscene letter to the mayor's daughter or the police chief's wife.

Or how about a letter expressing your true feelings to that nasty old aunt or uncle who might leave you something in his or her will?

Finally, with your clergyman, boss, local newspaper editor, or police chief in mind, there is always the possibility of a Polaroid camera with a delayed-shutter device, with which you could — well, since this is a family-rated book, I had better not elaborate on this particular option.

4: WHOM TO PLEDGE THINGS TO

If you choose to pledge money, possessions, services, or time to an organization, I think it is safe to say that the more you despise the potential recipient, the better your chances of losing weight successfully.

Therefore, unless there is some person or group you loathe with a livid passion (in which case your problem is a simple one), the potential recipient should be selected with great care.

To assist you, I have compiled a list of potentially hateful organizations. I say *potentially*. There is probably no cause or viewpoint imaginable, with the possible exception of preventing birth defects, that doesn't have at least two concerned organizations: one in favor of it and one opposed.

In Appendix A, I have listed 150 organizations, along with their addresses. If you can't find at least *one* to despise, there must be something wrong with you. (Or, dare I say, right with you.)

There are political organizations of every stripe, from farthest left to farthest right.

There are religious organizations from the most fervently pious to the most blatantly atheistic.

There are social organizations from those who want everything the way it was in 1892 to those who want worldwide revolution tomorrow.

There are organizations concerned with the military — from those who support it wholeheartedly to those who resist it with equal vigor.

And there are all manner of miscellaneous organizations, associations, and groups staunchly dedicated to the support, preservation, opposition, enjoyment, or elimination of virtually anything you can think of, from the return of the Russian czar to compulsory euthanasia to collecting used rosaries for the poor to legalizing marijuana to raising budgies.

In addition to these, you will find thousands more organizations listed in various books in the public library, most notably *The Encyclopedia of Associations* and *The World Almanac*.

Furthermore, there are 200-odd countries in the world. You could pledge a donation to the government of any one of them (the one you liked the least, of course) to be used for the general welfare of the citizenry.

There are tens of thousands of corporations and companies out there. Surely some are involved with goods or services that you believe have caused you or others harm.

Finally, there are thousands of high schools, colleges, and universities. At least one of them must have done something awful to you, your favorite team, or your daughter.

Whoever you choose, it might be wise to check and see if they accept donations. It is hard to imagine any who wouldn't, but it is conceivable that some may have general rules against accepting gifts — or, perhaps, some ethical concerns about manna coming, so to speak, through the back door, not to mention from someone who does not love them.

And no fair selecting an organization just because contributions to it are tax-deductible. If they happen to be, well I suppose you can claim the donation, but that somehow seems a bit like using your grand-mother's burial insurance for a trip to Hawaii.

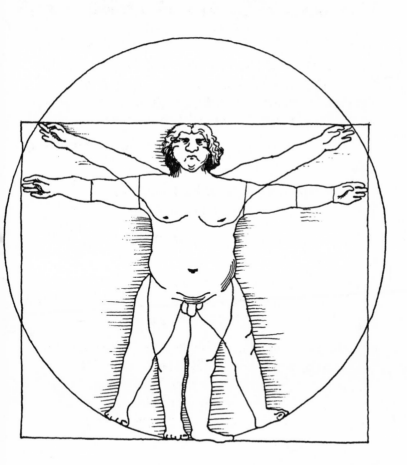

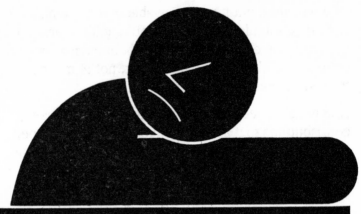

5: HOW TO SET YOUR WEIGHT-LOSS GOAL

Your goal for the self-blackmail period is best defined as weighing a certain number of pounds less than you weigh now. Realistically, of course, your absolutely perfect, ultimate, final weight is going to be a matter of appearance rather than what the scale says.

Given two ladies, each 5'6" tall and weighing precisely 130 pounds, you may well have:

— One 110-pound lady with 20 pounds of well-distributed muscles, and she looks great.

— One 110-pound lady with 20 pounds of ugly flab around her middle, and she looks terrible.

All this means is that your "final weight" — the weight you must reach in order to avoid the blackmail payoff, may *still* not be a logical stopping point.

Or, on the other, and far more pleasant to contemplate hand, you may actually lose *too* much, thereby requiring you to *gain* some weight after you reach your goal. (Is it not the secret dream of every fat person to have someone say, "My dear, you look positively *gaunt*"?)

Some people may wish to define their goal physically: fitting a certain garment, or achieving a given waist size, for instance. The imprecision of these measurements may cause problems, as any size 14 who has managed to squeeze into a size 12 dress will attest.

To help you decide on your final goal, you might wish to consult one of those standard insurance company charts showing the correct weight for every height. The various charts available are so different from one another that sometimes I wonder if the insurance companies have gotten their figures by sending people around to copy the charts from neighborhood drug store "no-springs honest-weight" penny scales.

One problem with these charts is that they usually need to know if you're large-boned, medium-boned, or small-boned. How is the average person supposed to figure this out without submitting to an autopsy — especially since we are told that some people who *look* big-boned are actually small, and vice versa?

And to further complicate matters, there are said to be people who have *some* big bones which are connected to *some* medium bones, which in turn may be connected to *some* small bones (now hear the word of the Lord).

The semi-final complication is age. People of the same sex, height, bone structure, and appearance can vary by as much as 20 pounds, depending upon their age.

And the final complication has to do with averages. Can you really be "over" weight if you weigh less than average? Well, yes, but only if 50 percent or more of the people in your height-age-bone category are fat, which is a real possibility.

At the end of this chapter, for those who feel comfortable staring at numbers on a chart, I have constructed a Weight Chart to End All Weight Charts: a composite of data from many sources. Use it if you must (although, as you will see, it is not excessively useful). I *do* think you'd do better deciding for yourself.

After all, the ultimate final decision on whether you've lost enough weight (or even too much weight) has to be made by you, yourself, with the aid of a precise scientific instrument.

It is called a mirror.

PSYCHOLOGICAL BACKGROUND

Caution. Not only is beauty in the eye of the beholder, so is almost everything else. People see what they *want* to see, or what they *expect* to see. In one classic experiment, people were quickly shown a picture in which a white man and a black man were squared off to fight. The white man held a straight razor; the black man was unarmed. When asked to describe the picture, most people, white and black, remembered that the razor was in the *black* man's hand, because that's what they *expected* to see.

In another experiment, most people who glance at this triangle

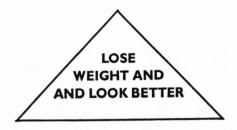

will not see the "obvious" mistake, because they don't expect to see words repeated in this fashion.

The relevance here is the problem of people seeing themselves in a way that no one else does. On one hand, a still-fat person may look so much better than he or she *used* to that the mind perceives thinness where there is still plumpness. On the other hand, there is the all-too-common situation in which the much-too-thin victim of anorexia nervosa genuinely sees herself as too fat. If you have concerns about your own objectivity, for goodness' sake, enlist the aid — and listen to the advice — of trusted friends.

Another word of caution. Do not bite off (so to speak) more than you can chew when you set your weight-loss goal. The only chance you'll have to adjust the amount of weight is *before* you sign the trust agreement.

So on one hand, you must not overdo it. Equally important, on the other hand you must not underdo it.

Case History #16:

Bill H. set a goal of 67 pounds in three months. Despite 89 days of near-starvation, he was still seven pounds away with 48 hours remaining. Fortunately, he knew a man who ran an all-night steam bath, where he sat for 47 hours, and he still needed a very short haircut and an enema to make the goal. All things considered, Bill felt it almost wasn't worth it. If he had it to do over again, he would have allowed five or six months.

Because people may get into situations like Bill's, I have included a section on Last-Minute Desperation Strategies, which may be found in Chapter 12.

Going too far on the side of caution can be even more unfortunate.

Case History #17:

Ginger C. vowed to lose 18 pounds in nine months. She did it with ease, but her boyfriend agreed with many others that she should have shed at least twice that much. Ginger, however, said she just couldn't face the psychological ordeal a second time, and now she goes through life displeasingly plump.

As a rule of thumb, then, your weight-loss goal should probably be somewhere between five and ten pounds per month. Any less is not enough to make it worth the agony of self-blackmail. Any more is likely to be unrealistically high.

The Weight Chart to End All Weight Charts

The factors included on this chart are your sex, height, age, and bone structure, as well as the average weight of all Americans, as reported by the U.S. government.

The first chart is for males, the second for females. The first column is your height. The next six columns show the average weight of Americans of that height, broken down by age range. (People who were otherwise broken down were presumably not surveyed.) The final three columns show the recommended weight range averaged from charts provided by three major life insurance companies.

As you can see, the ranges are quite large. A 5'4" woman, for instance, can be anywhere from 114 pounds to 154 pounds, depending on other factors. That's why this chart, and indeed, *all* charts, are not excessively useful — other than to help convince you, if you are off the chart *entirely,* that weight loss is called for.

All average and recommended weights are for naked people.

WOMEN

Height	Average weight for age: 18–24	25–34	35–44	45–54	55–64	65–74	Recommended weight for bone structure: Small	Medium	Large
4'10"	114	123	133	132	135	135	97–106	104–117	113–126
4'11"	118	126	136	136	138	138	98–108	106–118	115–129
5'0"	121	130	139	139	142	142	99–110	108–121	117–132
5'1"	124	133	141	143	145	145	101–113	110–124	120–135
5'2"	128	136	144	146	148	148	103–116	113–128	123–138
5'3"	131	139	146	150	151	151	106–119	116–130	126–142
5'4"	134	142	149	153	154	154	109–122	119–133	129–146
5'5"	137	146	151	157	157	157	112–125	122–136	132–150
5'6"	141	149	154	160	161	160	115–128	125–139	135–154
5'7"	144	152	156	164	164	163	118–131	128–142	138–158
5'8"	147	155	159	168	167	166	121–134	131–145	141–162
5'9"	150	158	162	172	170	169	124–137	134–148	144–165
5'10"	153	161	165	175	173	172	127–140	137–151	147–168

MEN

Height	Average weight for age:						Recommended weight for bone structure:		
	18–24	25–34	35–44	45–54	55–64	65–74	Small	Medium	Large
5'2"	130	139	146	148	147	143	121–127	124–134	131–143
5'3"	135	145	149	154	151	148	123–129	126–136	133–146
5'4"	139	151	155	158	156	152	125–131	128–138	135–149
5'5"	143	155	159	163	160	156	127–133	130–141	137–153
5'6"	148	159	164	167	165	161	129–135	132–146	139–157
5'7"	152	164	169	171	170	165	131–138	135–147	142–161
5'8"	157	168	174	176	174	169	133–141	137–150	145–165
5'9"	162	173	178	180	178	174	135–144	141–153	148–169
5'10"	166	177	183	185	183	178	137–147	144–156	151–173
5'11"	171	182	188	196	187	182	139–150	147–159	154–177
6'0"	175	186	192	194	192	187	142–153	150–163	154–181
6'1"	180	191	197	198	197	192	145–157	153–164	161–185
6'2"	185	196	202	204	201	195	148–161	154–171	165–190

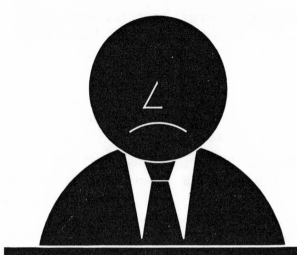

6: THE LEGAL DOCUMENTATION

Once you have chosen
- the nature of your self-blackmail,
- the potential recipient thereof, and
- your weight-loss goal,

you are ready for your legal document.

The legal aspects are, in most cases, refreshingly simple. A trust agreement is just a way to designate someone else (a trustee) to perform certain behaviors on your behalf.

The agreement does not *have* to be drawn up by a lawyer, but it's probably a good idea. The cost is relatively low. (My lawyer, who is not one of the world's cheapest, charged $75, including his service as a trustee, and the minimal time involved in terminating the trust at the end of the program.)

Since the whole *point* of the thing is to have an agreement that is as legally free of loopholes as possible, why take chances? If you suspect that you *may* be able to weasel out of an agreement, the temptation to do so, as time starts running out, may be irresistible.

If you make a simple money pledge, like mine, you could virtually copy my agreement (which appears in Appendix D) word for word, and you will have a valid, binding trust.

The agreement can be as simple or as complicated as you wish. This is a matter between you and your lawyer (or whoever draws it up).

The complications start entering in as you begin to ask yourself all kinds of "what if" questions. In my opinion, many of these are likely to be trivial, irrelevant, or worse yet, invitations to establish loopholes out through which you may be able to squirm. Some "what if's" may well be important for you, but I recommend using as few as possible.

Here are some "what if's" you may wish to consider:

1. What if I become ill during the weight-loss period?

You may wish the trust dissolved at this point, on the recommendation of a licensed physician — or you may wish the deadline extended by the length of time you were ill. Or you may not wish to include this eventuality at all. I know of no illnesses that require one to eat fudgey brownies, and I suspect it is pretty easy to lose weight while in a coma.

2. What if I have a debilitating accident?

By and large, the same arguments apply, except that it *is* possible to gain lots of weight while recuperating from a broken bone. Alas, I know from experience.

3. What if I become mentally ill?

Some people have suggested that you have to be mentally ill even to consider the Blackmail Diet in the first place. I choose to ignore these people. Mental illness is extremely hard to define, but if you worry about it a lot, you may be the sort of person who is susceptible. In this case, it should take a note from a psychiatrist (or perhaps a licensed clinical psychologist) to dissolve or suspend the trust.

4. What if I die?

Well, you'll sure lose weight then. But, as a matter of practicality, the trust should expire if and when you do.

5. What if I can't get to a doctor (or whoever is doing the final weighing) in time, at the end of the program?

If you are in a battlefield foxhole, or en route to the moon, you may indeed have problems. Either you can designate an alternative means of verifying your final weight, or you can figure that this one will be included in the "Catch All" clause, Clause Six.

6. What if the intended recipient of my pledge refuses to accept it?

If you have not cleared this in advance with the possible recipient, then an alternative should be named in advance, and included in the trust agreement. Under no circumstances other than meeting your weight-loss goal should refusal by the named recipients mean that your pledge is returned to you.

7. What if I am unable to make good on my pledge?

In other words, what happens if the money or goods are simply not available, or circumstances make it utterly impossible to perform the required labors? This is why goods or money should be put into a trust or escrow fund if at all possible, and why pledges of time or labor should be backed up by tangibles. However, if you *are* faced with this situation, you'll pretty much have to play it by ear.

Part of the solution depends on whether or not the named recipient chooses to sue you, as is their legal right, to recover whatever was promised.

However, if that which was pledged is irrecovably lost, stolen, or damaged, through no fault of your own, during the time the trust is in force, you should not be legally required to replace it, although you may feel a moral obligation.

8. What if gross irregularities are discovered?

What if it turns out that the initial weigh-in was inaccurate due to a defective scale? What if your doctor or lawyer turns out to be dishonest, perhaps even in the employ of the opposition? What if there are significant typographical errors in the trust agreement? There is no simple answer here. Clause Six may be relevant — or, since this *is* a legal document, its ultimate resolution may have to take place in a court of law.

9. What if something happens that could not possibly have been anticipated?

If we knew what they were, we could have listed them in advance, couldn't we? This is the "Catch All" clause, and I think it makes sense to include it *only* if you have a truly impartial and sensible trustee to interpret and enforce it. The clause (which appears in the sample trust agreement given in Appendix D) states that if, in the opinion of the trustee, something happens not within your control that prevents you from reaching your weight-loss goal, then the trustee has the right to void the trust and return the pledge to you.

This is risky, because it *does* leave a significantly large door *openable,* if not actually *open,* through which you can escape. This clause should be discussed with the trustee, who should clearly understand your wishes and his or her responsibilities in this regard.

Choosing a Trustee

Your trustee must be selected with much care and consideration. The wrong trustee can, for a number of reasons, hamper, subvert, or even sabotage your weight-losing effort.

The trustee is the person or organization charged with carrying out the terms and conditions of your trust agreement. Specifically, the trustee:

1. Holds the valuables, if any.
2. Determines whether or not you have met your weight-loss goal.
3. Determines whether or not there were any conditions or circumstances beyond your control which prevented you from reaching your goal.
4. Dispenses your valuables either to you or to the Other Party, or supervises the carrying out of the terms, if valuables are not involved.

Although a trustee may be virtually anyone — a relative, friend, lawyer, even a bank or a corporation — there are a variety of considerations that should be taken into account in choosing your trustee.

The single most important thing is that the trustee *not* be a friend or relative. The main reason for this has to do with number 3, above: the determination of special circumstances. Of course, for some people, number 1, holding the valuables, may be relevant. I know I've got a cousin or two I wouldn't trust with my carfare home, much less five thousand bucks.

A friend or relative may have a vested interest in preventing the forfeit of your valuables. If you even *suspect,* for instance, that your spouse would never really go through with it, it might make you careless.

Now to be sure, there may well be some circumstances that are *genuinely* beyond your control, where the decision of even a heavily biased trustee would never be questioned. I am unaware of any that have ever happened, but can envision some rare disease requiring a therapeutic diet that causes weight gain. Or being kidnapped by a crazed scientist who pumps chocolate sauce into your veins.

But most situations will be far less definitive.

Case History #18:

Julie P., desirous of losing 38 pounds, pledged her diamond engagement ring to the American Cancer Society. She named her husband Harvey, a foreman at a large cigarette factory, as trustee. She included the "Catch All" clause in her trust agreement.

When Julie failed to meet her goal, for no obvious reason, Harvey, acting as trustee, invoked Clause Nine, claiming that Julie had suffered extreme mental duress as the result of the illness of her canary, Budgie-Boy, and thus was exonerated from the terms of the agreement.

This clearly unethical use of Clause Nine is nonetheless legal, and Julie still wears her ring. She probably couldn't have gotten it off her pudgy finger anyway.

An impartial trustee, then, is far more likely to evaluate unforeseen events fairly, and thus to make the probability of such events occurring far less. (The case history of Magda R., reported in a supermarket weekly, who claimed that she was sprayed by a gas from a flying saucer which made her gorge herself on pasta, will not be given serious consideration here.)

So the best sort of trustee is someone who is neutral, impartial, and somewhat removed from involvement in the situation.

To avoid legal complications, if your trustee is a human being (as contrasted with a bank or corporation, that is, not with a chimpanzee), it is best to list an alternative human in case your first one dies, disappears, or is adjudged incurably insane — perhaps for having agreed to be a trustee in the first place.

You don't have to worry about this if your trustee is a bank, since banks rarely die and only occasionally go insane.

All things considered, an impartial lawyer is probably your best bet. If you don't know one, check the Yellow Pages under "Lawyers" or "Attorneys." Many cities have legal referral services.

Be sure you settle on a fee in advance. I have asked several lawyers what they would charge for drawing up a trust agreement and serving as a trustee, and have gotten a range of $25 to $150, with only one staid soul who was quite unwilling to become involved in something so far out of the mainstream of his legal practice. (He was fat, too.)

Once the terms of your trust agreement have been agreed upon, three copies should be prepared and signed by you and the trustee. One copy is yours, one stays with the trustee, and the third should be sent by certified mail (return receipt requested) to the party who will be the recipient of your pledge, should you fail.

The third is extremely important. When you send this signed or executed copy of the agreement, the other party is not only informed of what you are doing, but they can use the agreement as evidence in court, should you fail to keep your end of the bargain.

PSYCHOLOGICAL BACKGROUND

People are much less likely to do bad things if they believe they are likely to get caught, or otherwise pay for their sins. Two groups of 12-year-old boys were shown a filmstrip on the evils, dangers, and illegality of pornography. One filmstrip included a section on how "one-way" mirrors were used to spy on people; the other did not. Shortly after, each boy was left alone in a waiting room where there were some porno magazines visible in a partly open desk drawer. There was a large mirror on the wall. Of the boys who were told about one-way mirrors, only 7 percent opened the desk and looked at the magazines. Of the group that did not know about one-way mirrors, 81 percent looked.

If the potential pledge recipient *knows* about the pledge, the probability that there could be a messy and expensive law suit if you fail to make good is substantially larger. You increase the odds of "getting caught" should you try to escape from the trust.

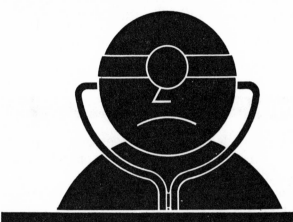

7: THE NECESSARY "SEE YOUR DOCTOR" REMARKS

Now that you are ready to begin, it is both necessary and desirable to warn you to see your doctor first.

Every diet book, magazine, article, and lecture warns you to see your doctor first.

These warnings are heeded by fat people just about as carefully and conscientiously as the warnings on cigarette packs are heeded by heavy smokers.

In other words, the vast majority of people about to embark on a diet never see a doctor. And most of them probably survive the ordeal anyway, just as most people who never fasten their seatbelts are still alive (at least for a while longer).

Nevertheless, it *is* a good idea.

So go see your family doctor and discuss the diet with him or her. You don't need to talk about self-blackmail if you'd rather not.

Of course, if you, like I, have a slightly tubby family doctor, the procedure may be a little embarrassing. Do it anyway. And pay your bill with a copy of this book!

PSYCHOLOGICAL BACKGROUND

How can there be any fat doctors, much less fat *diet* doctors? My wife once visited a well-known Beverly Hills cardiologist who specialized in weight control. The man was *fat*, and yet presumably his patients took his advice.

There is a peculiar phenomenon, discovered by communication psychologists, that the *content* of a message is remembered and believed, long after the *source* of the message is forgotten. In one experiment, two groups of subjects read newspaper articles on a new chewing gum. The articles were identical, except that one said the new product was Charles Manson's favorite gum to chew in prison; the other said it was the President's favorite gum to chew in the White House.

Soon after, the people who read the "Manson" article down-rated the gum, while the others rated it highly. But three months later, both groups rated the gum highly. The "Manson" readers had forgotten the source, but remembered the content of the message.

This helps to explain why rumors can be so deadly; why television commercials people "hate" still sell the product; and perhaps why fat diet doctors still have an audience. But it doesn't help explain *why* they are fat.

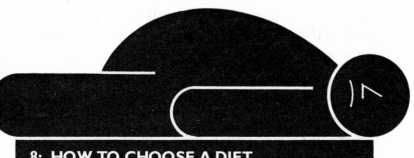

8: HOW TO CHOOSE A DIET

I am totally convinced that for the large majority of people (or, alternatively, for the majority of large people), *any diet whatsoever will work, as long as it is followed reasonably well.*

The main criterion for choosing a diet, then, should *not* be its alleged miracle quality — the thing that makes it different from all other diets in history — but rather whether it seems palatable, literally, to you.

Never mind that some formerly fat television personality lost 104 pounds on a diet of chocolate frappes and cabbage. If it doesn't appeal to you, you won't stay on it.

Never mind that a popular ladies' magazine rushes into print with "Our very own and very special goat's milk and chicken gravy reducing program." If you don't like the ingredients, you won't stick with the diet.

Never mind that the supermarket checkout stand weekly newspapers run what seems to be the same "miracle diet" plan every two or three weeks. If you don't like grapefruit and spinach, you won't lose 27 pounds in three days, or whatever they happen to be promising this week.

Never mind the latest paperback best-seller, which virtually guarantees that you'll lose "up to ten pounds a week" eating 28 snacks a day of apricots and hog jowls. If the eating pattern is alien to you, you won't follow it.

I happen to find it boring to stay on *any* diet for very long. But I *do* like to follow diets, rather than just try to eat less on my own.

So I have researched the subject, and come up with 127 different publicly available diets and other weight-losing schemes, programs, and methods.

Of course, I have not tried them all (it just *seems* that way!), but they all look reasonably OK to me. I make no guarantees, however, either as to their effectiveness or their safety for you, or for anyone. The only thing I can say with absolute certainty is that if for any reason any given diet isn't working for you, or isn't pleasant for you, by all means, abandon it and switch to another. And another. And another.

All the written diets have appeared in books issued by generally reputable publishers, or in well-known magazines. The various diet "clubs," such as Weight Watchers and T.O.P.S., have been around long enough to achieve respectability as well.

I most emphatically suggest that you do *not* stay on the same diet for your entire weight-losing period, or even most of it, *unless* it is, simultaneously

(a) very successful, and

(b) very enjoyable.

I have never found such a diet. If you know of one, for goodness' sake, write a book about it. I'll be the first to buy one.

If you prefer *not* to follow a diet, that's quite all right too. When you are on a self-blackmail program, the constant awareness of what could happen is like having a little guardian sitting on your shoulder going "No, no, no" every time you approach something that resembles food.

PSYCHOLOGICAL BACKGROUND

People get used to almost anything. A common experience is when there is a bad smell in the house. Soon, people in the house don't notice it any more, but others, just coming in, think it is awful.

This is even true of the ever-present fact of the terrible blackmail to be paid if you don't lose weight. Sometimes it is just too constant to serve as an all-day reminder. Even a tiny change in routine may help keep one alert to this factor. Some people wear their watch on the other wrist, keep their keys in a different pocket, or otherwise plant "unexpected" regular reminders that return their thoughts to the problem at hand, and possibly keep some food from entering the mouth.

I followed various diets at various times during my year of losing weight. They lasted anywhere from three days to about two weeks. I also went for as long as five weeks without paying close attention to my weight. (A goal that requires "only" six pounds a month allows for a lot of flexibility.)

Sometimes I used extreme measures (one of the 330-calories-a-day powders, or even short periods of fasting) to knock myself off stubborn plateaus — and in one case, as penance following a veritable eating orgy during the preparation of the food for the wedding of good friends. Even the threat of Dire Consequences, even the Guardian sitting on my shoulder, were not enough to keep me from licking the bowl wherein the double-fudge icing had lain. And I defy *any* human being to enter upon months of restrictive eating, and then resist a *large* and *heaping* bowl of grey Beluga caviar. I gained 7½ pounds that weekend.

The 127 diets are listed in Appendix B, along with their main claim to fame (grapefruit and spinach, weekly binges, low carbohydrate, no red meat, whatever).

The one thing I *don't* list is anything having to do with strenuous exercise, and the reasons for that are given in the following section.

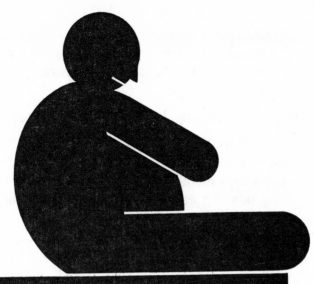

9: WHY I DON'T RECOMMEND EXERCISE

Jane Fonda and Richard Simmons may throw me off the softball team for this, but I honestly don't believe exercise plays any significant part whatsoever in the sort of weight-losing discipline that has been described.

Now quickly, before the Royal Canadian Air Force flies over and drops barbells on my roof, let me acknowledge that of course exercise *is* extremely valuable —

(a) to improve your appearance while, or after, losing weight (for instance, to prevent a spare tire around your middle); and

(b) to assist in losing weight (very, very slowly), or to help maintain weight after you've lost it.

But when it comes to a rigorous and dedicated program of concentrated weight loss, I submit that the difference between a conscientious exercise program and just loafing around doesn't amount to a hill of low-calorie sugar-free beans.

Consider the following:

Weight gain or loss is directly and precisely related to the number of calories you take in and use up. In general, when you take in 3,500 calories you gain one pound.

When you burn up 3,500 calories, you lose one pound.

(I am aware that some nutritionists believe that this can be somewhat different for some people, depending on their metabolic rates, the time of day they eat, the foods they eat, and even the order in which foods are eaten. But even if this turns out to be correct, the principle is the same: the more you eat, the more you gain, and vice versa.)

It really doesn't much matter where the calories come from.

You eat one large, rich, gooey chocolate fudge cake and you gain one pound.

You eat 29 large heads of lettuce and you gain one pound.

Doing nothing whatsoever uses up about 25 to 30 calories per hour (just to keep your body warm, your heart pumping, and other internal functions going). So if you stayed in bed 24 hours a day, doing nothing whatsoever (including eating!), it would take a normal person four or five days to lose a pound. (Fat people often have faster metabolic rates, and grossly overweight people on total fasts have actually lost as much as a pound a day while lying in a hospital bed.)

Now, at the other end of the exercise spectrum, let us consider a vigorous game of full-court fast-break basketball. That uses up about 550 calories per hour. So, in order to lose a pound while charging up and down the court, going elbow-to-elbow with Dr. J. and his friends, you'd have to play continuously for six hours and 22 minutes, no time outs.

Thus, to lose an ambitious amount like ten pounds a month, you could either

(a) lie in bed for 30 days doing nothing, or

(b) play 105 vigorous games of basketball.

All right, all right, before everybody jumps on me, I am well aware that there are shortcomings to this line of reasoning. But my basic point, I think, is valid:

It takes so much vigorous exercise to lose a significant amount of weight, and it is so simple to lose weight without exercise, that exercise may just not be worth the effort.

PSYCHOLOGICAL BACKGROUND

Quite apart from the physiological factors discussed in the text, there is the matter of the difficulty of doing two new and complicated things at once. Jokes were made about one recent president who "couldn't walk and chew gum at the same time."

There is evidence that trying to learn two unrelated new behaviors at the same time may be far more than twice as hard as just learning one. For example, subjects in one experiment were divided into two groups. One group was told to memorize the Gettysburg Address and then to write it down from memory. Then they practiced pressing buttons in a certain order when different colored lights flashed. The second group was interrupted regularly by the lights-and-buttons routine while they were memorizing and writing the Address. The second group took about three times as long to both write the speech and press 100 buttons as the first group.

Many people have experienced the problem of having two big events going on at the same time: a family fight and an important exam at school; planning for a trip and preparing for a business meeting.

It is often very hard to keep the two things apart. For some people, then, the pain, learning, and preparation of getting into an exercise regimen may well interfere with the concentration and dedication required for the weight-loss program. Do the exercise, sure, but perhaps *after* you're well along on the weight losing.

The following chart demonstrates how much of a whole lot of things you would have to do in order to lose ten pounds. The times, distances, and amounts are approximate, because some people run or make beds or whatever with more vigor than others. Use this chart to help decide what if any activities to concentrate on as part of your exercise program. And don't feel guilty at all if you defer exercising regularly until *after* you are well along on your diet.

Activity	Hours of this activity necessary to lose 10 pounds	Amount of this activity necessary to lose 10 pounds
Fast running	40	300 miles at top speed
Fast swimming	40	2,500 laps of big pool
Running up stairs	44	Up the Empire State Building 22 times
Fast bicycling	60	New York to Chicago at top speed
Shoveling snow	70	Driveway 1/2 mile long
Sawing wood	70	Sawing a 2 × 16,800 in half the long way
Skiing	80	Down the Matterhorn 1,400 times
Tennis (singles)	80	240 sets
Tennis (doubles)	100	300 sets
Making beds	120	1,400 beds
Bowling	140	560 lines
Golf	140	990 holes
Cutting grass	140	30 acres, hand mower
Mopping floors	180	Mop a room 10 feet wide and 1 mile long
Taking a bath	350	1,000 long baths
Brushing teeth	350	318 times a day for 1 month
Cooking	350	Carving 3,040 turkeys
Reading	400	59 Michener books
Playing the piano	470	2,634 Rachmaninoff concerti
Playing cards	700	5,608 hands of gin rummy
Singing	700	"Star-Spangled Banner" 14,128 times
Driving a car	700	New York to Boston 176 times
Watching television	1,400	"Laverne & Shirley" every week for 93 years

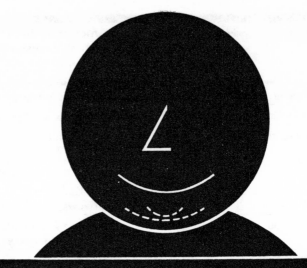

10: HOW TO DIET SUCCESSFULLY

As you undoubtedly know from past experience,
losing weight is an incredibly boring thing to do.
It seems to take forever, and it is gastronomically
boring as well. Even the "diet gourmet" recipes all
start tasting the same by the end of the second week.
Day-to-day progress is literally impossible to see. A
242-pound human doesn't look any different from a
241-pound human, no matter how much blood, sweat,
and tears went into removing that one pound.

In the absence of the rewards of really good food, it
can be extraordinarily useful to institute a series of
short-term rewards and satisfactions. They can make
the entire process very much more bearable.

Here are seven things that have worked for me, to
make the entire procedure more interesting, and
perhaps even contribute to weight loss. If they don't
seem right for you, ignore them. But I do think a few
of these, or similar kinds of things you devise for
yourself, can be a big help.

A series of little, short-term rewards or encourage-
ments have been shown to speed up various learning
processes. In one experiment, for instance, volun-
teers were divided into three groups. Each group
was given an identical task: putting together a large
jigsaw puzzle. Each group worked in a different
room. One group worked without interruption. The
second group worked in a room into which people
came every 15 minutes, apparently on other business. The "interrupters" stopped to look, and said
things like, "Gee you're doing a great job," or "It's
really going faster than any other group we've had."
The third group was similarly interrupted, but every
5 minutes.

The experiment was repeated many times. The
average time for finishing the puzzle for Group 3 was
72 minutes, for Group 2, 90 minutes, and for Group
1, 117 minutes. The more rewards, the faster the
goal was achieved.

In another experiment, hungry rats were timed as
they learned to run through a maze. One group found
tiny bits of food at various points along the maze,
when they made a correct turn. The other group got
an equal amount of food, but all of it at the end of the
maze. The learning times of the first group were
significantly shorter.

Many little rewards, in addition to or instead of one
big one, seem to have a positive effect.

---

1. Frequent Weighings
I am well aware that many diet books and experts tell
you to weigh yourself only once a week, if that often.
Nonsense! If you could weigh yourself every three
hours, that would not be often enough. Every time
you learn your weight, it is either a little reward or a

little penalty—and in either event, it serves to spur you on to better things until the next weighing.

Of course, weight fluctuates during the course of a day. Every time you drink a big glass of water, you weigh almost a pound more—for a short while. So you mustn't panic or grow distressed by these fluctuations, especially if the general direction is downward.

The more accurate your scale, the more often it makes sense to weigh yourself. I am quite convinced that I could not lose weight at all without a good scale. I am not 100 percent certain of this, but I have a strong suspicion that the scale itself actually removes weight. The fat sinks down through the toes, right into the scale. You see, it is most assuredly the case that when I weigh myself morning and night (and any other time I happen to be padding by the bathroom with no clothes on), I lose weight. When I don't, I usually don't.

Furthermore, the more accurate the scale, the more I lose. It could well be that the small reward and encouragement of even a four-ounce loss (which wouldn't even show up on an ordinary bathroom scale) provides sufficient motivation for being careful and good until the next weighing-in. (Remember, only four ounces a day means, in but three years, a 274-pound loss!)

So we bought a junior version of those balance-beam scales you see in doctors' offices. About $100 from a mail-order catalogue. It weighs accurately in quarter-pound gradations, which is close enough. I would be happier with a scale that weighed in hundredths of an ounce. If I had such a scale, however, the problem is that every time I moved my bowels, had a haircut, shaved extra close, or rubbed some dirt off my elbow, I'd probably be rushing off to weigh myself and see the effect.

2. The Chart

I believe it is important to chart your progress. The ritual of daily (or at least very regular) changing of the chart reinforces the reward (or punishment) factor. It can be slightly (or even extremely) satisfying, or it can be a "grit your teeth and vow to do better tomorrow" sort of experience.

The more elaborate the chart, and the more often it needs your attention, the better.

My chart was hung prominently in the dining room, where I could see it from my place at the dining table. It consisted of four sets of numbers hanging on little nails, sort of like the numbers used on non-electronic scoreboards.

Every day, then, I adjusted the numbers to tell the world, and remind myself, how many pounds I had lost, how many pounds remained to be lost, how many days had elapsed, and how many days were left.

There was also a graph on which I plotted my daily loss or gain, and there was an "information line" which reminded me whether or not I was "on schedule," "ahead of schedule," or "behind schedule." It looked like this:

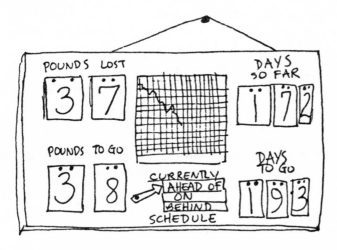

I strongly recommend having a chart, and urge keeping it up to date every single day — although my dear wife knows that I did not follow this good advice myself. When I suspected or knew that I had gained weight, I somehow forgot to adjust the chart. But with it staring me in the face at every meal, I could not ignore it for long. I was never more than three days late.

3. Telling People What You Are Doing

It may be quite helpful (and unfailingly interesting) to tell people exactly what you are up to. Not just that you are trying to lose weight, but that you have entered into a self-blackmail scheme, and all the grisly details thereof.

If you simply announce that you are trying to lose weight, some close friends may be supportive, most people couldn't care less, and there are always a bunch of others that seem to have been sent by the devil himself to talk you out of it ("Oh, come on, just a little mashed potatoes can't hurt . . .").

I once observed this phenomenon in its ultimate form when a Jewish Mother met a Famous Faster. A friend who is a civil rights lawyer was defending Dick Gregory before the U.S. Supreme Court. The friend invited his mother — quite possibly the original Jewish Mother — to meet Gregory in the Supreme Court cafeteria. The Mother was aghast to see that Gregory was not eating. He explained that he was two weeks into a 30-day fast, protesting the mistreatment of Native Americans.

The sweet old lady had never *heard* of such a thing. So Gregory launched into a long and detailed lecture on the moral and philosophical basis for fasting; its role in history; the importance of Gandhi and his followers; what it meant to him, and why he was doing it. When he finished, she put her hand solicitously on his arm and said, "Yeh, but maybe you'll eat just a *little* something."

If, however, you tell people (even Jewish Mothers) about your self-blackmail, they seem to go out of their way to help you. A minister, aware of my pact with the Nazis, actually snatched a plate of chocolate cake from my hands one afternoon — and I guess I was rather glad that he did.

4. Arrange to See People You Haven't Seen for a While

While you can take pleasure in a tiny loss as reflected on your scale, there is no visual pleasure in attempting to observe a four-ounce loss in the mirror. There is, however, immense joy in seeing people you haven't seen for a while, and basking in their reaction.

This is the case even if you engineer a "chance" meeting specifically for that purpose.

After months of back-breaking, nerve-wracking, stomach-rending dieting, I "ran into" Richard Crews, whose first words were, "Say, you've lost a little weight, haven't you?" Thanks, Dick.

5. Amaze Yourself (the Roast Beef Method)

So this lady went into the meat market and asked the butcher for a 12¾-pound roast beef. He sawed one off, but it only weighed 11½ pounds. "It won't do," she said, "it has to be 12¾." He tried again. 12¼ pounds. "Won't do." Finally, on the fourth try, he hit it on the nose. "Shall I slice it," he asked, "or will you take it whole?" "Oh, I don't want to *buy* it," she replied. "I just wanted to see how the weight I've lost looks."

You should consider doing the same. Or, rather, almost the same. Maintain a bag, box, or suitcase that weighs precisely the amount you have lost to date. Keep adding sand, rocks, chopped liver, or whatever to adjust the weight as you lose. Keep it in plain view. Look at it often. Heft it. Marvel over the fact that you used to lug that much weight around with you day and night. Better still, carry the suitcase around with you for at least an hour a week.

I enjoy bowling. When I had lost 16 pounds, I found it astonishing that I had been carrying an extra bowling ball, so to speak, around with me constantly. Now that I am about five bowling balls lighter, I find it almost impossible to conceive of having carried five bowling balls everywhere I went.

6. Promised Splurges

It is, of course, traditional for us serious dieters to promise ourselves a Big Splurge upon reaching some interim goal: the first ten pounds, the halfway point, etc.

However, based on several cases (including my own), I find a curious phenomenon that seems to set in when on a self-blackmail program. Reaching the Splurge Criterion seems to bring about a feeling that perhaps it could be delayed just a little longer. Like the child who keeps saying, "Just ten minutes more, please," and saying it every ten minutes, the self-blackmailer may well find him or herself saying, "Well perhaps I'll just wait another ten pounds before I. . . ."

There is clear evidence that experimental subjects perform most tasks better when there is a clear goal and a well-defined reward. Subjects in one experiment were asked to see how long they could hold their breath. One group simply held their breath as long as they could. They averaged 38 seconds. The second group was told that their goal was one minute, and they sat watching a big clock as they held their breath. Their average time was 57 seconds. The third group also was given the one-minute goal, and promised five cents for each second over one minute they lasted. Their average time for holding their breath was 72 seconds.

Finally, what are we to make of the fourth group, which was given a goal and a reward — and a "rigged" clock that ran one-third slower than it should? These people lasted an average of what they *thought* was 62 seconds, which was, in reality, 83 seconds! Mind over matter.

My first planned splurge was to have been at 20 pounds. I thought about it every day for weeks. I was like a middle-aged kid on his first visit to Santa Chef: "An' a pepperoni pizza, giant size, an' a chocklit fudgy sundae, an' a 32-ounce sirloin, an' a Lobster Newburg an'. . . ."

But when I reached that point — well, it's hard to explain, but it just didn't seem quite as necessary as I had thought. Ten more pounds, I thought, and then I'll enjoy it so much more. And then ten more. And ten more. And so on. And then I was only ten pounds from the goal.

Let me hasten to reassure you that my taste buds haven't withered and died and that my stomach hasn't shrunk to the size and usability of an old prune. Upon emerging from the doctor's office with the letter attesting to the fact that I had met my goal, I headed directly for Clown Alley, whereat I downed three large Polish sausage sandwiches and a large chocolate shake. Four hours later, I had a big, steamy bowl of spaghetti. An absurd seven pounds in six hours. Took me two weeks to get back to my goal weight. And yes, of course it was worth it.

7. Incriminating and Embarrassing Evidence

I think it is a good idea to have photographs of yourself taken before you begin. You may not wish to look at them — in fact, I strongly recommend that you do not — but there will come a time when you'll be glad you have them, and may even be displaying them to your friends, not unlike a proud grandparent (except that instead of the arrival of eight pounds, you'll be displaying the departure of a good deal more).

A minor but knotty problem is how to get the "before" pictures taken without suffering undue embarrassment. It is bad enough to be fat underneath lots of protective clothing (where no one can see that you're really fat, right???) — but to be fat in a bathing suit in front of others is much more threatening.

So I bought one of those delayed-action timer gadgets for my instant camera, but it never worked right. When I got any pictures at all, they were either of (a) my back, as I was walking away from the camera, or (b) my nose, as I was leaning forward to see why it hadn't gone off.

I actually toyed with the idea of removing some of my garments in a coin-operated photo machine, but I couldn't think of what I would say to the (a) policeman or (b) sweet old lady who would, without fail, come along at precisely the wrong 1/50th of a second.

Finally I bit the bullet (no calories there) and went into the local professional photography studio. Stephen Gillette may have thought I was a nut case, but at least I was willing to pay. My one small concession to sanity was refusing to take delivery of the photos until I was 50 pounds lighter. Then I could be (and was) well and truly disgusted. Good work, Stephen!

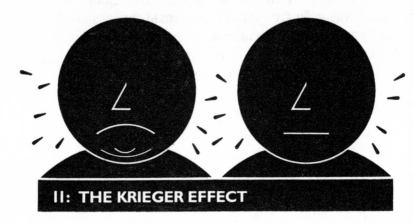

II: THE KRIEGER EFFECT

An interesting side effect to the self-blackmail technique has been noted. I have called this phenomenon the Krieger Effect, since it was first observed and reported by one Harold Krieger, who personally experienced it.

Mr. Krieger is a Formerly Plump Person. Even though he is of normal dimensions now, he still has to watch his weight rather carefully.

Aware of my self-blackmail program from the start, Mr. Krieger noticed that he has not only become much more conscious of his own eating patterns because of thinking about *my* program, he also believes he has actually lost weight through worrying about whether or not I would reach my goal.

This suggests that overweight persons who may be surrounded by *other* overweight friends and relations (which is frequently the case) may actually help these associates lose weight during a self-blackmail program.

Three variations on the notion of the group effect have been proposed:

1. All Pay, but Only One Diets

In this version, two or more fat people contribute to a common pot (or, perhaps more kindly, kitty), but only one of the group would be required to lose weight in order to prevent the funds from going to an organization disliked by all. The hope here is that others in the group would be spared the mental anguish of a self-blackmail program of their own, while still possibly losing weight due to the Krieger Effect.

2. All Pay, All Diet, All Cooperate

Two or more people contribute equally to the kitty, and all embark on a self-blackmail diet program. The rule here is that everyone in the group must meet his or her goal, or *everybody's* money is forfeited. What an immense amount of moral support there would be here, not to mention the possibility of overt action if one of the group seems to be faltering. (Watch out for Krazy Glue added to the toothpaste!)

3. All Pay, All Diet, All Compete

Here we have a scenario in which two or more highly competitive fatties each put an equal amount — preferably a *sizeable* equal amount — into the kitty, and all set realistic and mutually acceptable goals. But now, instead of the money going to some outside organization, the rule is that the money in the kitty is shared equally among all group members who meet their goal. What a cutthroat venture this might become, especially if you had, say, a few dozen participants to the tune of a thousand or more. Ideally, the participants would dislike each other as well, which would make the incentive to lose the weight, not the money, even greater. (How long before someone establishes a business as a Blackmail Diet Plan Broker, bringing together members of such a consortium? No, you, not me. I'm too busy. But let me know if you do it, so I can put it in the next edition of this book.)

PSYCHOLOGICAL BACKGROUND

There is all kinds of evidence that one's psychological state can have a dramatic effect on physical behavior.

For instance, we observe serious and somber bankers who "go wild" in the enthusiasm of an exciting football game, or meek and timid people who turn into vigorous heroes when confronted with a burning building or a crime in progress.

It is well known that concern or fear can cause biological changes: nausea, diarrhea, flushed skin, etc. Anger or extreme distress can bring the digestive action of the body to a halt. So it may not be surprising that worry and concern could alter the metabolism, or otherwise help control weight.

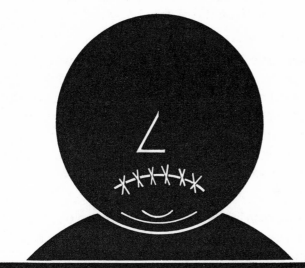

12: DESPERATION CITY: EMERGENCY PROCEDURES YOU DON'T EVEN WANT TO THINK ABOUT

Some people may find themselves in one of two desperate situations: either the dilemma of simply being unable, for whatever reason, to lose weight, despite the spectre of a major penalty; and/or of having very little time left, and a fairly substantial amount of weight yet to lose, in order to avoid the dire consequences.

Of course, one should never have gotten into this situation in the first place. But that doesn't help one bit after it has happened (or is happening). Here are some desperation measures that could conceivably be considered.

When You're Unable to Lose Weight

Two techniques have been used by truly desperate fat people: jaw-wiring, and the blind loop. And there's something new on the distant horizon that may offer hope to us all.

Jaw-wiring is, quite simply, having the jaws wired shut, so that the teeth cannot move far enough apart to permit solid food to enter. The technique is simply rendered by oral surgeons. Of course it is still possible to suck a lot of calories in through a straw, but it is much less likely to happen. When desired, the jaws can be unwired as easily as they were wired in the first place.

The blind loop is the popular name for an operation technically called a jejuno-colostomy. Normally performed only on people at least 100 pounds overweight, the operation consists of severing nearly all (up to 20 feet) of the lower bowel, and sewing the ends together, so no food can enter it. With only a couple of feet of functional bowel remaining, most food just passes on through unabsorbed; just enough is absorbed to keep you functioning.

The two advantages are that you can eat all you want and never gain weight — and the operation is surgically reversible if you wish to return to internal normality.

The two disadvantages are that nearly all people with blind loops have permanent diarrhea and average three or four bowel movements a day; and that *any* abdominal surgery is going to be both expensive and risky.

The faint hope is a new substance, being tested on human beings as we speak, that purports to coat the inside of the intestine with a temporary coating that does not permit food to be absorbed. While the coating is in place, you can eat anything you want without gaining. It sounds like a temporary blind loop, with none of the hazards or discomforts. The inventors say that if all goes well, they hope to have it on the market before 1990, and no, they don't need any more human guinea pigs; I tried.

What about acupuncture, acupressure, hypnosis, psychotherapy, prayer, diet pills, and injections of hormone made from the urine of pregnant women? All these have apparently worked on a short-term basis for some people. I think it especially advisable to consult a doctor before embarking on any of these programs (except perhaps prayer, and if that works, why are most television evangelists on the plump side?).

When You Need to Lose a Lot, and Fast

Do not abandon hope. You mustn't count on this in advance, but it *may* be possible to lose as much as ten pounds (even more for some people) in as short a time as two or three days.

The art, or perhaps science, of instant massive weight loss evolved because of the needs of those two classes of sportsmen who have to meet rigid weight limits: boxers and jockeys. As these people well know, the weight loss isn't necessarily permanent, but when faced with a "weigh-in" deadline, the only real need is to weigh that much at that moment in time.

Here, then, is an assortment of last-minute emergency procedures. Some are clearly more desperate than others. Which you might consider would depend on how much you have to lose — both in weight, and in the consequences of your pledge. Some of the procedures may seem quite trivial, and indeed they are, representing loss of only a fraction of an ounce. But a few grams here, a few grams there, it all adds up. Wasn't it that noted plump person, Ben Franklin, who said something like, "Take care of the ounces and the flab will take care of itself"?

1. Fasting

The object is to eat *nothing whatsoever.* Nothing. If you can stand it, let not even a drop of water pass your lips. If you are in good health, you can do this for two days with no danger of physical harm. If you become desperate for something, chew on an ice cube. A small low-calorie ice cube.

Abstaining from everything for 48 hours can mean a loss of as much as five to seven pounds — most of it liquid loss, which needs to be replaced later. Take a multi-vitamin pill if you wish, but you'll live without it.

Warning: Don't ever fast beyond two days without medical permission or supervision. You can do all kinds of permanent harm to your system.

---

2. Sweating

You want to remove as much liquid as you can from your body. Sweating (or, if you are delicate, perspiring) is a good way to do this. You'll know from experience what makes you sweat best: exercising in heavy clothes, sitting in a steam bath, taking a sauna, or whatever. The body is capable of exuding perspiration at the rate of up to a quarter of a pound per hour. By the time you are ready for the Mr. Prune Look-Alike Contest, you could be up to ten pounds lighter. (A major-league baseball pitcher once told the press that he lost eleven pounds during each nine-inning game — and then, not unexpectedly, gained it all back over the next three days.)

3. Laxatives and diuretics

It normally takes two to three days for food to go from one end to the other, so to speak. To speed up the process, and to be sure there is no excess baggage hanging around in your intestines, you may wish to consider a *one-time* use of a laxative. Again, you'll know what works best for you.

Diuretics speed up elimination of liquids from the body, and there are over-the-counter non-prescription brands available at drug stores.

Neither of these items can have any benefit whatsoever to a sensible, regular weight-loss regimen, and both should be avoided except in emergency situations.

4. Crying and spitting

Empty your tear ducts if you can. If you can cry at will, cry at will. If you cannot cry at will, think deeply on what it will mean if you don't make your goal. Or simply peel and slice onions.

Expectoration (the polite word for spitting) is an often-overlooked means of removing liquids from the body. Experimentation (never mind how) has shown that continuous spitting can produce from six to eight ounces of product per day.

5. Removal of hair

Depending on how fuzzy you are, all the hair on your body, from the top of your head to the soles of your feet (in the case of fat vampires) weighs anywhere from under four ounces to more than a pound.

6. Finger and toenails, nose-blowing, ejaculation, etc.

A little here, a little there, it all adds up.

7. Removal of internal parts

Well, it seems pathologically dumb even to contemplate, but as I have discussed the desperation situation with people, the topic has arisen. It has been suggested that there could be situations where removal of a non-vital organ (appendix, tonsils, gall bladder, etc.) might be perceived as better, somehow, than the penalty for not meeting the goal.

8. *Removal of external parts*
Arms weigh about 10 pounds, legs weigh about 20 pounds, and if you take this seriously, I suggest you may wish to begin with the head (about 14 pounds).

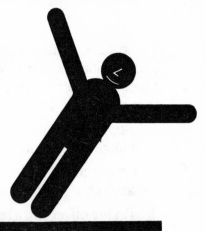

13: STAYING THIN
THROUGH SELF-BLACKMAIL

Every diet book and diet program I've ever encountered has a section on the Importance of Restructuring Your Eating Habits; the Building of Life-Long Good Food Habits in order to stay thin.

I say *hogwash.*

I concede that this notion may have merit for some peole. But I am not one of them. And I don't believe I've ever met anyone who is.

Oh, sure, people give lip service to the idea. They may even have the best of intentions. But the proof, as they say, is in the putting: the putting on of weight again, that is. As mentioned earlier, 98 percent of people who lose weight put it back on again within two years.

I hereby publicly acknowledge, once and for all, that

1. I will *never, ever* have sensible eating habits. I fully intend to spend the rest of my life eating erratically.

2. I fully intend, with equal vigor and determination, never to be fat again. And this time (yes, of course I've said that line before), I am going to back up my determination with another self-blackmail program, to be certain I will not gain.

To be sure, at times I may choose to eat reasonably and sensibly, perhaps even for days or weeks at a time. But at other times, and I can predict they will be in the majority, I fully intend to do things like:

1. Skipping four meals in a row, and then eating all of a huge and gigantic pepperoni pizza.
2. Eating celery for breakfast, celery for lunch, and a large chocolate cream pie for dinner.
3. Taking off an extra ten pounds on a crash gimmick diet, and then gaining it all back in one glorious all-day binge.
4. And so on.

Fortunately, I have a wonderfully understanding wife, who only occasionally says things like, "Don't you think you may be ruining your gastro-intestinal tract?"

Well, maybe. Except for this: I figure that over the next 30 years, I will be consuming approximately 33,000,000 calories.

On one hand, that represents 30 years' worth of three well-balanced meals per day. On the other hand, it represents 66,938 large bowls of ravioli, or 82,108 butterscotch milkshakes (thick), or 108,196¾ pieces of Church's fried chicken — or even 29 years and 364 days worth of total starvation followed by 196,428 tacos on the final day.

I may not do it. But I reserve the right.

The one thing I know for sure is that I cannot keep weight off without help. I know that I am extremely prone to gaining it all back again. I know that I have done it twice. Since I first got fat more than 20 years ago, I have lost a lot of weight three times, keeping it off for about three years once, and about eight months the second time. Both times, I relied on my common sense, integrity, intelligence, and willpower. Total failure.

And so I reluctantly but necessarily admit that I need the "crutch" of another, long-range self-blackmail scheme in order to keep the weight off. That is what I am doing. Here are the details.

The basic philosophy of the Maintenance Blackmail Program is that payment of some kind would be required if your weight rose above some predetermined level.

There are two different ways to go about this: the graduated pledge, and the all-or-nothing pledge.

The Graduated Pledge

For this kind of self-blackmail, you must choose as a pledge something that can be subdivided into small parts, like money, or hours of your time, rather than something that is indivisible, like a car or a painting.

You set your base weight — where you want to stay — and then pledge a certain amount of whatever for every pound you are above that weight on a regularly scheduled weigh-in.

___

Case History #19:

Carla K. reached her desired weight of 125 pounds in plenty of time to avoid any penalty. Immediately, she undertook a maintenance plan, whereby she agreed to come in to her doctor's office during the first ten days of January, May, and September each year for a weigh-in. For every pound over 125 that she weighed at these times, her trustee was required to send $100 to the John Birch Society, a staunchly conservative organization which Carla roundly despised.

Carla considered both more frequent and less frequent weigh-ins, but concluded that three per year was right for her. Any more often would be inconvenient; any less often and there would be the temptation to "bal-

loon up" and then have to "balloon down" during the
interim periods.

All of the considerations of choosing a pledge, a recipient, a trustee, etc., discussed in detail in Chapters 2 to 5, are equally relevant here, too.

The All-or-Nothing Pledge

The circumstances here are almost identical, but in this case, the entire amount of whatever was pledged would go to the Other Party upon the *first* transgression.

Again, there should be regular weigh-ins — at least twice a year — but if you even once exceed your limit, by even one pound, you lose the whole works.

This option is, of course, much more extreme than the Graduated Pledge, and should only be entered into by persons with a long history of failing to maintain weight loss. Like me.

Case History #20:

John Bear, an author, wrote a book called The Blackmail Diet. *Sales of this book produce royalty payments, which are paid by the publisher, Ten Speed Press, twice a year, on March 31 and September 30.*

Bear has entered into a contractual agreement with Ten Speed Press as follows: each year, between March 16 and 31, and again between September 15 and 30, Bear must appear at the premises of Ten Speed Press, with his Detecto Model 1600-B bathroom scale (the model top-rated by Consumer Reports*), or equivalent. In normal outdoor clothing, but without shoes, he must display a weight of less than 180 pounds to an officer of Ten Speed Press.*

If Bear fails to appear, or if his weight is above 180 pounds, all the royalties that would have been paid to him from the sale of The Blackmail Diet *for that half-year time period are to be paid, instead, to the Invisible Empire Knights of the Ku Klux Klan.*

This, in some respects, is not a typical agreement, since most people don't have royalty contracts, and very few of those who do have royalty contracts have a publisher nutty enough to go along with something like this. (Can you imagine walking into the Harvard University Press with your little bathroom scale under your arm? I may have to ask Marina to knit me a scale cozy, anyway. . . .)

Therefore, I have engaged a lawyer to draft a standard, all-purpose sort of Maintenance Blackmail Trust Agreement, which is reproduced in Appendix D.

PSYCHOLOGICAL BACKGROUND

Quite possibly the major obstacle in establishing and sticking with a maintenance plan is that most Americans and Canadians seem incapable of long-range planning. Psychologists who are concerned with national cultural types, or "modal personalities," tend to say that one of the main distinguishing features that separates Russians from many Western people is their ability to establish and live with Five-Year Plans, Ten-Year Plans, Twenty-Year Plans, and so on.

When you are brought up not to expect things to change for the better tomorrow or next week, you are probably much better able to think about a weight-maintenance agreement that could stretch well into the next decade. Now the only question is, why are there so many fat Russians?

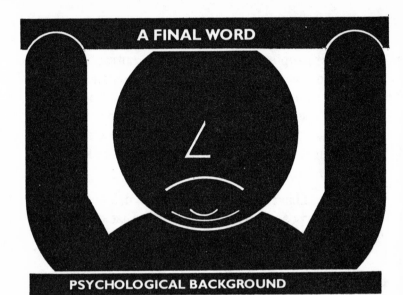

A FINAL WORD

PSYCHOLOGICAL BACKGROUND

In the Introduction, I promised that there would be no cheery inspirational messages, and so there will not. Let me leave you, then, with these few psychological insights.

Most people who think about self-improvement or bettering themselves or their lot in life never do anything about it other than think about it and read about it.

The majority of people who buy those best-selling books on finance and investment never invest a dime. Most of the people who buy those best-selling exercise and work-out books never get beyond the third week. When I surveyed 1,000 buyers of my book, *How to Get the Degree You Want,* a year after their purchase, I found that 15 percent were pursuing a degree, 10 percent had decided not to, and 75 percent were "still thinking about it."

That last category is the key. Thinking about it. It is very hard on the self-image for a person to admit that he or she will *never* be rich, fit, degreed, or non-fat. So there is always that feeling that "someday, someday. . . ." These people keep buying self-improvement books, and even starting in on programs of various kinds. "See, I'm really trying," they think they're saying. "I haven't given up yet."

Sadly, most of them *have* given up. Given up everything but buying the books and magazines that make good fantasy reading. "What if I really *did* get fit, make money, go back for my degree, clear up my complexion, attract men (or women or who-or-whatever you want to attract), find true happiness and inner peace, make a killing in the magnesium futures market, and/or lose weight." Well, that's all very nice, but unlikely to happen while you're sitting there reading.

The whole practice of psychiatry, clinical psychology, counseling, and newspaper advice columns is based on the assumption that if people come to understand their problems, they may be able, with professional guidance, to act on them. The mere fact that you have gotten as far as this page demonstrates that your interest level is high. The Blackmail Diet is a psychologically valid method to take advantage of your current (but sure to fade) enthusiasm, and make it virtually impossible to turn back.

Good luck, and let me know how you do.

John Bear
Ten Speed Press
P.O. Box 7123
Berkeley, California 94707

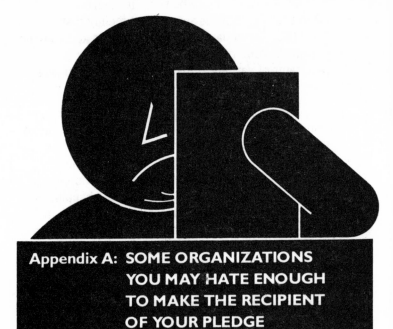

Appendix A: SOME ORGANIZATIONS YOU MAY HATE ENOUGH TO MAKE THE RECIPIENT OF YOUR PLEDGE

All of these are legitimate, genuine organizations, and the probability is high that all would be delighted to receive your pledge should you fail to meet your weight-loss goal. Both the categories and the selection of organizations are quite arbitrary, but surely there is *something* here for everybody to hate.

Race and Civil Rights

American Nazi (National Socialist White People's) Party, 2507 N. Franklin Rd., Arlington VA 22201

Congress of Racial Equality, 1916 Park Ave., New York NY 10037

Ku Klux Klan, Invisible Empire Knights, Box 700, Denham Springs LA 70726

Southern Christian Leadership Conference, 334 Auburn Ave. N.E., Atlanta GA 30312

Stop Forced Busing, Box 133, South Boston
MA 02127

Anti-Apartheid Movement, 13 Selous St., London
NW1, England

South African Tourist Corporation, 610 Fifth Ave.,
New York NY 10020

National Association for the Advancement of Colored
People, 186 Remsen St., Brooklyn NY 11201

National Association for the Advancement of White
People, Box 10625, New Orleans LA 70101

Operation PUSH (Jesse Jackson), 930 E. 50th St.,
Chicago IL 60615

National States Rights Party ("patriotic white
racist"), Box 1211 Marietta GA 30061

Sex and Decency

Johns and Call Girls Against Repression, Box 1011,
Brooklyn NY 11202

The Moral Majority, 305 Sixth St., Lynchburg
VA 24504

Adult Film Association of America, 1654 Cordova St.,
Los Angeles CA 90007

Coyote (for decriminalization of prostitution), Box
26354, San Francisco CA 94126

The National Federation for Decency, Box 1398,
Tupelo MS 38801

Childhood Sensuality Circle (sex for children), Box
5164, San Diego CA 92105

Mistresses Anonymous, Box 151, Islip NY 11751

Women Against Pornography, 358 W. 47th St., New
York NY 10036

SIECUS, The Sex Information Education Council of
the U.S., 80 Fifth Ave., Suite 801, New York
NY 10011

Religion (and the Lack of It)

American Atheist Women (Madalyn Murray O'Hair), Box 2117, Austin TX 78768

American Bible Society, 1865 Broadway, New York NY 10023

World Council of Churches, 150 Route de Ferney, CH-1211, Geneva 20, Switzerland

Freedom from Religion Foundation, Box 750, Madison WI 53701

Messianic Jewish Alliance (Jews for Jesus), Box 1055, Havertown PA 19083

Campaign for Surplus Rosaries, 1821 W. Short 17th St., North Little Rock AR 72114

Society for the Study of Evolution, Campus Box B-334, University of Colorado, Boulder CO 80309

Society of Evangelical Agnostics, Box 515, Auberry CA 93602

American Humanist Association, 7 Harwood Dr., Amherst NY 14226

Spiritual Counterfeits Project, Box 2418, Berkeley CA 94702

War and Peace

War Resisters' League, 339 Lafayette St., New York NY 10012

Veterans of Foreign Wars, VFW Bldg., Kansas City MO 64111

Committee Against Registration and the Draft, 201 Massachusetts Ave. N.E., No. 111, Washington DC 20002

Daughters of the American Revolution, 1776 D St. N.W., Washington DC 20006

National Interreligious Service Board for Conscientious Objectors, 550 Washington Bldg., 15th & New York Ave. N.W., Washington DC 20005

Association of the U.S. Army, 2425 Wilson Blvd., Arlington VA 22201

Bertrand Russell Peace Foundation, Bertrand Russell House, Gamble St., Nottingham NG7 4ET, England

Crime and Punishment

Friends of the FBI, 1835 K St. N.W., Suite 600, Washington DC 20026

National Coalition Against the Death Penalty, 138 Tremont St., Boston MA 02111

Prisoners' Union, 1317 18th St., San Francisco CA 94107

Society of Former Special Agents of the FBI, 2416 Queens Plaza S., Long Island City NY 11101

Abortion and Family Planning

Americans Against Abortion (Billy James Hargis), 5800 E. Skelly Dr., Tulsa OK 74135

Planned Parenthood Federation of America, 810 7th Ave., New York NY 10019

National Abortion Rights Action League, 1424 K St. N.W., Washington DC 20005

Zero Population Growth, 1346 Connecticut Ave. N.W., Washington DC 20036

Nuclear Power

Campaign for Nuclear Disarmament, 24 Great James St., London WC1N 3EV, England

Institute of Nuclear Power Operators, 1820 Water Place, Atlanta GA 30339

Karen Silkwood Fund, 1324 N. Capitol St.,
Washington DC 20002

Society for the Advancement of Fission Energy, Box
353, Monroeville PA 15146

Nuclear Weapons Freeze Campaign, 4144 Lindell St.,
Suite 404, St. Louis MO 63108

Concerned Citizens for the Nuclear Breeder, Box
208, Ruffsdale PA 15679

Environment and Ecology

The Sierra Club, 530 Bush St., San Francisco
CA 94108

International Snowmobile Industry Association, 7535
Little River Turnpike, Suite 330, Annandale
VA 22003

Save the Redwoods League, 114 Sansome St., Suite
605, San Francisco CA 94104

National Forest Products Association, 1619
Massachusetts Ave. N.W., Washington DC 20036

American Rivers Conservation Council, 323
Pennsylvania Ave. S.E., Washington DC 20003

Communism and Anti-Communism

Communist Party of the U.S.A., 235 W. 23rd St., 7th
Floor, New York NY 10011

John Birch Society, 395 Concord Ave., Belmont
MA 02178

Forum for U.S.-Soviet Dialogue, Box 19289,
Washington DC 20036

Anti-Communist League of America, 3100 Park
Newport, Suite 101, Newport Beach CA 92660

Anarchist Association of the Americas, Box 840, Ben
Franklin Station, Washington DC 20044

Arabs and Jews

World Jewish Congress, 1 Park Ave., Suite 418, New York NY 10016

Campaign to Save the People of Palestine, 1825 Connecticut Ave. N.W., Suite 211, Washington DC 20009

American Jewish Alternatives to Zionism, 133 E. 73rd St., Suite 404, New York NY 10021

Jewish Defense League (Meir Kahane), 34 W. 38th St., 6th Floor, New York NY 10018

Guns

National Coalition to Ban Handguns, 100 Maryland Ave. N.E., Washington DC 20002

National Rifle Association of America, 1600 Rhode Island Ave. N.W., Washington DC 20036

Suicide

International Association for the Prevention of Suicide, 1811 Trousdale Dr., Burlingame CA 94010

American Euthanasia Foundation, 95 N. Barth Rd., Suite 301, Ft. Lauderdale FL 33304

Smoking

Tobacco Institute, 1875 I St. N.W., Suite 800, Washington DC 20006

National Cancer Foundation, 1 Park Ave., New York NY 10016

Drinking

American Temperance Society, 6840 Easter Ave. N.W., Washington DC 20012

American Beverage Alcohol Association, 10 E. 40th St., Suite 2000, New York NY 10016

Men and Women

National Organization for Women, 425 13th St. N.W., Suite 1048, Washington DC 20004

Men's Equality Now, Box 189, Forest Lane MN 55025

Mormons for the ERA, 5520 N. 32nd St., Arlington VA 22207

Civil Liberties

American Civil Liberties Union, 132 W. 43rd St., New York NY 10036

Conservatives Against Liberal Legislation, 3124 N. 19th St., Suite 5, Arlington VA 22201

Campaign for Economic Democracy (Jane Fonda/Tom Hayden), 409 Santa Monica Blvd., Suite 214, Santa Monica CA 90401

Black Silent Majority Committee, Box 5519, San Antonio TX 78201

Playboy Foundation, 919 N. Michigan Ave., Chicago IL 60603

Public Citizen (Ralph Nader), Box 19404, Washington DC 20036

Phenomena

Amalgamated Flying Saucer Clubs of America, Box 39, Yucca Valley CA 92284

Vampire Research Center, Box 252, Elmhurst NY 11373

American Society for Psychical Research, 5 W. 73rd St., New York NY 10023

American Federation of Astrologers, Box 22040, Tempe AZ 85282

Committee for the Scientific Investigation of Claims of the Paranormal, 1203 Kensington Ave., Buffalo NY 14215

Automotive

National Committee to Repeal the 55 MPH Speed Limit, 310 Emelie St., Collinsville IL 62234

Center for Auto Safety, 1223 Dupont Circle Bldg., Washington DC 20036

Motor Vehicle Manufacturers Association, 300 New Center Bldg., Detroit MI 48202

Motorcycle Industry Council, 2400 Michelson Dr., Suite 110, Irvine CA 92715

Japan Light Machinery Information Center, 1221 Ave. of the Americas, New York NY 10020

Punks, etc.

Parents of Punkers, Box 4830, Long Beach CA 90004

Better Youth Organization (pro-punk), P.O. Box 67A64, Los Angeles CA 90067

Hell's Angels (their phone is 415/550-9280, but I was afraid to call and ask for the address)

Homosexuals

Gay Rights National Lobby, Box 1892, Washington DC 20013

Caucus of Gay, Lesbian and Bisexual Psychiatrists, 245 E. 17th St., New York NY 10003

Custody Action for Lesbian Mothers, Box 281, Narberth PA 19072

Food

Overeaters Anonymous, 2190 W. 190th St., Torrance CA 90504

National Association to Aid Fat Americans ("Fat can be beautiful"), Box 43, Bellerose NY 11426

North American Vegetarian Society, Box 72, Dolgeville NY 13329

American Meat Institute, Box 3556, Washington DC 20007

Potato Chip/Snack Food Association, 1735 Jeff Davis Hwy., Suite 903, Arlington VA 22202

Drugs

National Organization for the Reform of Marijuana Laws, 2036 P St., Suite 401, Washington DC 20036

Potsmokers Anonymous (anti-marijuana), 316 E. 3rd St., New York NY 10009

Neo-American Church (pro-LSD), Box 450, Redway CA 95560

International Narcotic Enforcement Officers Association, 112 State St., Suite 1310, Albany NY 12207

Metrification

American National Metric Council (pro-metric), 5410 Grosvenor Lane, Bethesda MD 20814

Americans for Customary Weight and Measure (anti-metric), 47 West St., New York NY 10001

Traditional Politics

Democratic National Committee, 1625 Massachusetts Ave. N.W., Washington DC 20036

Republican National Committee, 310 1st St. S.E., Washington DC 20003

Animals

American Cat Fanciers Association, Box 203, Pt. Lookout MO 65726

American Kennel Club, 51 Madison Ave., New York NY 10010

American Budgerigar Society, 2 Farnum Rd., Warwick RI 02888

American Anti-Vivisection Society, 801 Old York Rd., Suite 204, Jenkintown PA 19046

International Council Against Bullfighting, 13 Graystone Rd., Tankerton, Whitstable, Kent CT5 T54, England

International Organizations

The United Nations Association, 300 E. 42nd St., New York NY 10017

The Trilateral Commission, 345 E. 46th St., New York NY 10017

The Club of Rome, 23, Viale Civitta del Lavoro, I-00144, Rome, Italy

The Irish Question

American Aid to Ulster (pro-British), Box 42, Philadelphia PA 19105

American Committee for Ulster Justice (anti-British), 129 Third St., New City NY 10956

Labor and Management

American Management Association, 135 W. 50th St., New York NY 10020

AFL-CIO, 815 16th St. N.W., Washington DC 20006

National Right to Work Legal Defense Foundation (anti-union), 8081 Braddock Road, Suite 600, Springfield VA 22160

United Farm Workers of America (Cesar Chavez), La Paz, Keene CA 93531

Americans Concerned about Corporate Power, Box 19312, Washington DC 20036

One of a Kind

Academy of Television Arts and Sciences, 4605 Lankershim Blvd., Suite 800, North Hollywood CA 91602

Accordion Federation of North America, 11438 Elmcrest St., El Monte CA 91732

All Russian Monarchist Front, 65 E. 96th St., New York NY 10028

American Association of Dental Victims, 3320 E. 7th St., Long Beach CA 90804

American Council of Spotted Asses (the animal, I think), 2126 Fairview Place, Billings MT 59102

American Indian Movement, 1209 4th St. S.E., Minneapolis MN 55414

Association for the Preservation of Anti-Psychiatric Artifacts, Box 9, Bayside NY 11361

Bald Headed Men of America, 4006 Arendell St., Morehead City NC 28557

Casket Manufacturers Association of America, 708 Church St., Evanston IL 60201

Church of Monday Night Football, Box 2127, Santa Barbara CA 93102

Committee to Form a U.S.-Albanian Friendship Association, Box 8238, Chicago IL 60680

International Brotherhood of Old Bastards, 2330 S. Brentwood Blvd., Suite 666, St. Louis MO 63144

International Flat Earth Society, Box 2533, Lancaster CA 93539

Lefthanders International, 3601 S.W. 29th St., Topeka KS 66614

Mothers-in-Law Club International, 420 Adelberg Lane, Cedarhurst NY 11516

National Apartment Association (landlords), 1825 K St. N.W., Washington DC 20006

National Association of Civil Service Employees (bureaucrats), 7185 Navajo Rd., Suite C, San Diego CA 92190

Neurotics Anonymous International, Box 4866, Cleveland Park Station, Washington DC 20008

Non-Circumcision Educational Foundation, Box 37, Appalachin NY 13732

Richard III Society, Box 217, Sea Cliff NY 11579

Scrooge: Society to Curtail Ridiculous Outrageous and Ostentatious Gift Exchange, 1447 Westwood Rd., Charlottesville VA 22901

Society of Dirty Old Men, Box 18202, Indianapolis IN 46218

127

None of these diets is being endorsed. They are presented to show the incredible variety of approaches offered by the diet writers of America. All of them have probably worked for some people at some time, at least for a while. Try one, try 'em all, or do whatever else you want — as long as you meet your goal and don't have to forfeit your pledge.

The summaries given are very brief, and may not reflect all the ramifications of the given diet. When there are multiple authors, only the first is given. Many of the books could easily fit in more than one category, but they are listed only in what seems to be the most relevant one.

High Carbohydrate

Doctor Rechtschaffen's Diet for Lifetime Weight Control and Better Health.
Joseph S. Rechtschaffen, M.D. Random House, New York, 1980.

Low-fat, low-cholesterol, strict regimen for four weeks, then flexible high-carbohydrate, high-residue diet.

Doctor Solomon's Easy No-Risk Diet.
Neil Solomon, M.D. Coward McCann & Geoghegan, New York, 1974.

1,200 calories a day, rigorous lists to follow, high carbohydrates, low protein, modest fat. A best-seller.

The Thin Game — Diet Scams and Dietary Sense: A Unique, Easy to Follow Program for Permanent Weight Loss.
Edwin Bayrd, Newsweek Books, New York, 1978.

High carbohydrates, medium fat, low protein, some walking.

Low or No Carbohydrates

The Astronaut's Diet.
Malcolm Smith, D.V.M. In *Rating the Diets,* Consumer's Guide, Skokie IL, 1975.

The former veterinarian who supervised astronauts' nutrition proposes 1,250 calories, no sweets, no alcohol, careful portion control, much variety.

Doctor Atkins' Diet Revolution: The High-Calorie Way to Stay Thin Forever.
Robert C. Atkins, M.D. David McKay, New York, 1972.

No carbohydrates, all the fat you want (butter, mayonnaise, cheese, etc.), never count calories. A best-seller.

The Drinking Man's Diet.
Gardner Jameson. Cameron, San Francisco, 1964.

Eat or drink what you want as long as it contains less than 60 grams of carbohydrates a day.

The Lazy Lady's Easy Diet — A Fast Action Plan to Lose Weight Quickly.
Sidney Petrie. Parker Publishing, West Nyack NY, 1969.

Low carbohydrates, smaller portions, and psychological tips.

The Miracle Diet for Fast Weight Loss.
'Sidney Petrie. Parker Publishing, West Nyack NY, 1970.

Low carbohydrates, low fat, high protein, natural foods, and six meals or snacks a day, within a 600 to 1,200 calorie range.

The New York Times Natural Foods Dieting Book.
Yvonne Young Tarr. Quadrangle Books, New York, 1972.

Low carbohydrates, and make them honey, fruit, and whole wheat bread. Avoid processed foods.

Slimming Down.
Ed McMahon. Grosset & Dunlap, New York, 1972.

The famous sidekick tells how he lost weight eating 250 calories a day worth of carbohydrates.

Sweet and Dangerous.
John Yudkin. Peter H. Wyden, New York, 1972.

Suggests low carbohydrates, low sugar, high fat, and high protein.

High Protein

Boston Police Diet and Weight Control Program.
Sam S. Berman, M.D. Dell Publishing, New York,
1974.

High protein, high fat, low carbohydrates, and a
recommended thyroid extract pill. Disavowed by the
Boston Police Department.

A Chicken for Every Pot: The Chicken Diet.
Rudolph E. Noble, M.D. Delphi Books, 1980.

Two chicken meals a day, preferring white meat to
dark; it has less than half the calories of beef, a third
those of pork.

The Complete Scarsdale Medical Diet and Dr.
Tarnower's Lifetime Keep-Slim Program.
Herman Tarnower, M.D. Rawson, Wade Publishers,
New York, 1978.

Almost unlimited fruits and vegetables, and "plenty"
of meat. A best-seller.

Doctor Carlton Fredericks' Low Carbohydrate Diet.
Carlton Federicks. Award Books, New York, 1965.

High protein, pretty high fat, don't count calories, and
eat six meals a day.

Doctor Stillman's 14-day Shape-Up Program.
Irwin M. Stillman, M.D. Delacorte Press, New York,
1974.

High protein, some carbohydrates, and up to ten
glasses of liquids a day.

The Doctor's Quick Weight Loss Diet.
Irwin M. Stillman, M.D. Dell Publishing, New York,
1968.

Lots of protein, since it takes more energy to digest
it, and "raise the fires" of metabolism. All you want of
lean meat, fish, eggs, poultry, and at least eight
glasses of liquid a day. A best-seller.

You Can Be Fat-Free Forever.
Dr. L.M. Elting and Dr. Seymour Isenbert. St. Martin's Press, New York, 1974.

Lots of meat, little fruit and vegetables, three prunes or a slice of cranberry jelly a day, eight big glasses of water, and that's all.

Low Protein

The Doctor's Quick Inches Off Diet.
Irwin M. Stillman, M.D. Dell Publishing, New York, 1970.

No meat, poultry, or fish, high vegetables and fruit. In six weeks' use, the diet "pulls extra fat from between the muscles."

Jeanne Jones' Food Lovers Diet — A Safe, Sane, Way to Stay Thin Forever.
Jeanne Jones. Charles Scribner's Sons, New York, 1982.

All you want of almost anything except animal proteins.

High Fiber

The Beverly Hills Medical Diet.
Arnold Fox, M.D. Bantam Books, New York, 1981.

Fiber-laden and unrefined starchy foods plus stress-free eating, to replace stress with zest.

Bircher-Benner Keep-Slim Nutrition Plan.
Staff of the Bircher-Benner Clinic. Nash Publishing, Los Angeles, 1973.

Low- or non-fat diets, heavy on fruit and muesli, plus some exercise.

Doctor Siegal's Natural Fiber Permanent Weight Loss Diet.
Sanford Siegal, M.D. Dial Press, New York, 1975.

Naked calories (no nutritional value) are the culprit. Sound nutrition plus nine heaping tablespoons of bran a day.

The High Fiber Way to Health.
Carlton Fredericks. Award Books, New York, 1965.

Lots and bran and other fiber, some meat, low-calorie portions.

The Save Your Life Diet.
David Reuben, M.D. Random House, New York, 1975.

High fiber, low calorie, lots of roughage, much bran flakes, honey, and molasses.

Diets Requiring Exercise

Diet Is Not Enough.
Irving B. Perlstein. Collier, New York, 1972.

All the lean meat you can eat, no drugs, regular exercise, and get your personal life together.

Fit or Fat—A New Way to Health and Fitness Through Nutrition and Aerobic Exercise.
Covert Bailey. Houghton Mifflin, Boston, 1978.

Aerobics plus high carbohydrate and good proteins, no fats, to develop athletically trained muscles.

How Sex Can Keep You Slim.
Abraham I. Friedman, M.D. Prentice-Hall, Englewood Cliffs NJ, 1972.

Sex not only uses up calories, but helps keep your mind off food.

The Pritikin Program for Diet and Exercise.
Nathan Pritikin. Grosset & Dunlap, New York, 1979.

The diet is low in fat, cholesterol, protein, and sugar; high in starches; and lots of walking.

The 200 Calorie Solution.
Martin Katahan. W. W. Norton, New York, 1982.

Small meals throughout the day, and enough exercise to burn off an additional 200 calories a day, which will result in a loss of 20 pounds a year.

The West Point Fitness and Diet Book.
Col. James Anderson. Rawson Associates, New York, 1977.

Exercise programs for all ages, low fat, no desserts, and a food exchange program (substitutions from supplied lists).

The Whole Life Diet—An Integrated Program of Nutrition and Exercise for a Lifestyle of Total Health.
Thomas J. Bassler, M.D. M. Evans, New York, 1979.

No fads, balanced foods, and jogging, running, or aerobics.

Precise Calculations

Calories In, Calories Out—The Energy-Budget Way to Fitness and Weight Control.
James Leisy. Stephen Greene Press, Brattleboro VT, 1981.

Calculating your own body's fat content and metabolic rate, then matching what goes in to the expenditure of calories, carefully calculated.

The Carbo-Calorie Diet.
Donald S. Mart. Doubleday, Garden City NY, 1973.

A long list of foods with their carbo-calorie rating, calculated from a special formula involving carbohydrate and calorie counting.

The Computer Diet.
Vincent Antonetti. M. Evans, New York, 1973.

Many computer-generated diets, and an immense number of charts and tables.

The Digital Dieter's Handbook.
M. de Ville. Hartford Publishing, Denville NJ, 1973.

Diet based on the ratio of protein to calories. One follows their lists rigorously and drinks lots of water.

Doctor Abravanel's Body Type Diet and Lifetime Nutrition Plan.
Elliot Abravenel, M.D. Bantam Books, New York, 1983.

Calculate which of four body types you are, and based on that, select the appropriate diet and lifetime nutrition plan.

How to Get Thinner Once and for All — The Revolutionary and Medically-Proven Get-It-Off Keep-It-Off PFI System.
Morton B. Glenn, M.D. E. P. Dutton, New York, 1965.

Relearn how to eat, through portion frequency item control. Diet selection charts based on sex, height, age, amount overweight. Rigid diets. No pork, prunes, bagels, cherries, grapes, much else.

The Revolutionary 7-Unit Low Fat Diet — Direct from London.
Jean Carper. Rawson, Wade Publishing, New York, 1981.

Count nothing but Fat Units (charts are supplied), and eat 7 a day. Range is from 0 (spaghetti, much else) to 141 (cheesecake).

Natural Food Diets

Doctor Van Fleet's Amazing New Non-Glue-Food Diet.
Dr. Van Fleet. Parker Publishing, West Nyack NY,
1974.

No foods that have been altered during the manufacturing process; high on unsaturated fats.

Folk Medicine.
D. C. Jarvis, M.D. Fawcett Crest, Greenwich CT,
1958.

The big best-seller craze of the late '50s is based on a high-potassium diet with lots of apple cider vinegar.

*Lose Weight Naturally: Prevention Magazine's
No-Diet No Willpower Method.*
Mark Bricklin. Rodale Press, Emmaus PA, 1978.

Count calories carefully, exercise, use natural foods only, and pay attention to the Nutrient Value/Calorie Density Ratio of foods.

The Natural Way to Super Beauty.
Mary Ann Crenshaw. David McKay, New York, 1974.

Using the "four friends," which are cider vinegar, lecithin, kelp, and Vitamin B-6.

The Weighing Game and How to Win It.
O. and D. Riccio. Rodale Press, Emmaus PA, 1974.

High protein, organic foods, unsalted nuts, and six small meals a day.

Dairy Products

The Ice Cream Diet.
Gaynor Maddox. Award Books, New York, 1970.

Six small eatings a day, four of them ice cream, totaling 1,000 calories.

The New Diet Does It.
Gayelord Hauser. Berkley Medallion Books, New York, 1972.

A quart of yogurt a day, high protein, and lots of green and yellow vegetables.

Oil-Based Diets

Calories Don't Count.
Herman Taller, M.D. Simon & Schuster, New York, 1961.

Even though the author of this super best-seller of the early '60s was convicted of mail fraud for claims made, many people swore that they *could* lose weight on 5,000 calories a day by eating the right fats and a dose of safflower oil before every meal.

Doctor Cantor's Longevity Diet.
Alfred J. Cantor, M.D. Parker Publishing, West Nyack NY, 1967.

Based on the "Cantor cocktail" (safflower oil and diet soda), plus fish, greens, lots of water, no baked goods except angel food cake.

Eat and Become Slim.
Hirohisa Arai. Shufunotomo, Tokyo, 1972.

Japanese best-seller diet with lots of vegetable oil, no animal oil, fried rice, fried chicken, Chinese foods.

Extremely Low Calorie

Cambridge Diet Plan.
Cambridge International, Monterey CA.

Utilizes a diet food developed by a Cambridge University physician, whose research alleges that 330 perfectly balanced calories a day is sufficient in two-week sessions, with normal low-calorie eating in between. Available through local Cambridge Counselors. Similar products with names like "The University Diet" are sold in health food stores.

Acupressure

Dr. Bahr's Diet — The 10-Second-a-Day Acupressure Reducing and Diet Book.
Frank R. Bahr. Morrow, New York, 1978.

Identifies points on the body whose stimulation is said to reduce hunger drive. Ear lobes are a traditional one. A newly discovered point on the inside of the upper lip. Combined with a high-protein, low-carbohydrate, no-fat diet.

Fasting

Doctor Linn's Last Chance Diet.
Robert Linn. Lyle Stuart, Secaucus NJ, 1976.

Modified fast, with nothing but a protein supplement of predigested animal protein, four to eight ounces a day.

Fasting, the Ultimate Diet.
Allan Cott. Bantam Books, New York, 1975.

The logistics and dangers of short- and long-term total fasts as part of a diet plan.

How to Get Well.
Paavo Airola. Health Plus Publishers, Phoenix AZ, 1974.

A weight-reduction and health-improving plan involving fasts of one to two weeks (some juices only), plus daily enemas.

The Zero Calorie Diet.
Shana Alexander. *Life* magazine, October 11, 1963.

A careful look into the benefits and dangers of the total fast.

Prepared Foods

How to Stay Slim and Healthy on the Fast Food Diet.
Judith Stern. Prentice-Hall, Englewood Cliffs NJ, 1980.

Basis is one fast-food meal a day, with tips on keeping their calories down ("hold the mayo," a vanilla rather than a chocolate milkshake, etc.).

I Hate to Cook Diet.
Deborah Blumenthal. *Mademoiselle* magazine, April 1982.

A balanced low-calorie diet entirely from foods requiring no preparation, straight from the supermarket shelf and freezer.

Switching from One Diet to Another

The Berkowitz Diet Switch — The Miracle Diet for the 80's.
Gerald M. Berkowitz, M.D. Arlington House, Westport CT, 1981.

Six basic diets. Plan is to change from one to another every few weeks (high protein, one big meal a day, fill up on salads, six small meals a day, etc.).

Controlled Cheating—The Fats Goldberg Take It Off, Keep It Off Diet Program.
Larry Goldberg. Doubleday, Garden City NY, 1981.

Eat anything you want one day a week (eventually every third day). Must not ever change the day. Goldberg also has declared Kansas City a free food zone, and on his annual trips there gorges himself, gaining up to 20 pounds in a week, then losing it promptly at home. (I identify with this philosophy more than any other listed here.)

The Freedom Diet—Games Dieters Play.
Leslie Jane Maynard. Frederick Fell, New York, 1977.

Select daily menu from specific portions in 12 different groups, including ice cream and cookies. Lots of behavioral change advice.

The Last Best Diet Book.
Joyce Bockar, M.D. Stein & Day, New York, 1980.

Psychiatrist offers behavioral techniques, with binge-and-starve cycles. Her diet includes fried egg whites, fish or chicken, no fruits or vegetables, no flour.

Slimming the French Way.
Albert Antoine. G. P. Putnam's Sons, New York, 1956.

French best-seller based on seven-day cycles of seven diets: vegetable day, meat day, egg day, milk day, fish day, fruit day, normal day. Two eight-week sessions of this three months apart. Based on proper portions of ingredients, smaller portions, few liquids (except on milk day).

Behavioral Modification Diet Programs

Act Thin, Stay Thin—How to Lose Weight and Keep It Off.
Dr. Richard B. Stuart. W. W. Norton, New York, 1978.

The psychological director of Weight Watchers offers behavioral tips to develop self-control as the major factor.

The Anti-Diet—The New Pleasure-Power Way to Lose Weight.
Lynn Donovan. Nash Publishing, Los Angeles, 1971.

Since dieting is nothing but rules, we have vicarious pleasure in breaking those rules. Once one learns why one gets hungry, it is possible to stop being so without diet.

Break Out of Your Fat Cell—The Holistic Mind-Body Guide to Permanent Weight Loss.
Jeane Eddy Westin. CompCare Publications, Minneapolis MN, 1979.

Develop non-condemnatory, self-assertive, self-actualizing attitudes while you diet, to reduce guilt, increase coping behaviors.

Breaking the Diet Habit—The Natural Weight Alternative.
Janet Polivy. Basic Books, New York, 1983.

No diets, but pay attention to body's natural signals to learn and reach your natural weight; evolve into eating just what you need.

Diets Don't Work—A Breakthrough Discovery: The Secrets of Losing Weight Step by Step When All Else Fails.
Bob Schwartz. Breakthru Publishing, Galveston TX, 1982.

Dozens of questionnaires, applying the principles he learned in *est* to behavioral modification.

Eating Is Okay — The Behavioral Control Diet.
Henry A. Jordan, M.D. Rawson Associates, New
York, 1976.

It's not what, but how and why we eat that counts.
Understand inner drives and life patterns, keep
detailed diaries, graphs, and charts, eat slowly, leave
food on the plate, etc.

*The Expense Account Diet — How to Lose Weight on
$24.95 a Day.*
Jonathan Dolger. Random House, New York, 1969.

Train yourself to eat dietetically in fancy restaurants
on elegant food. Order appetizers as the main course,
etc.

From Fat to Skinny.
Lawrence Reich, M.D. Wyden Books, 1977.

Fantasy eating. Get good enough at eating high-
calorie food in your fantasies and you won't need to in
person.

How to Be a Thin Person.
Raysa Rose Bonow. Random House, New York,
1977.

Obesity is a learned addictive behavior disorder,
which can be treated. Keeping a journal of all you eat
is the start of the treatment.

*How to Eat Like a Thin Person — The Dieter's
Handbook of Do's and Don'ts.*
Lorraine Dusky and J. J. Leedy, M.D. Simon &
Schuster, New York, 1982.

Little theory and great amounts of practical tips for
getting through each day.

The Love Diet — The Way to Permanent Weight Control.
John Janset, M.D. Collier Books, New York, 1978.

Someone else takes over your food entirely: orders it, buys it, cooks it, serves it. You are not allowed to do anything but eat what you are given.

A Minnesota Doctor's Guide to Weight Reduction and Control.
John Eichenlaub, M.D. Prentice-Hall, Englewood Cliffs NJ, 1977.

Emphasis on eye appeal and behavioral tips (the practical, sensible North Country approach).

The O.K. Way to Slim — Weight Control Through Transactional Analysis.
Frank Laverty, Grove Press, 1977.

Fatness is programmed in early childhood. We have a "fat script" we follow. Therapy suggested to discover and correct behavioral patterns.

The Southampton Diet — The Diet That Keeps the Beautiful People Thin, Beautiful, Super-Active.
Stuart Berger, M.D. Simon & Schuster, New York, 1982.

A psychiatrist who once weighed 420 pounds tells how to change mental patterns, use mood-controlling foods, stay happy, eat lots of vegetables.

The Stick to It Diet Book — The First Truly New Idea Ever.
Bernard Geis Associates, 1971.

Lots of little stickers with reminder messages to put around the house, on the refrigerator door, etc.

The Thin Book by a Formerly Fat Psychiatrist.
Theodore Rubin, M.D. Trident Press, New York,
1966.

Behavioral tips only, but suggests a high-protein,
low-carbohydrate diet. Emphasis on philosophy that
some is better than lots. If you can't help bingeing,
then make it a modified binge. Half a milkshake is
better than finishing it.

*Winning the Losing Battle — Why I Will Never Be Fat
Again.*
Eda LeShan. Thomas Y. Crowell, New York, 1979.

Any diet will work if you stay on it. The psychological
factors are the most crucial.

Changing the Metabolism

*The Bio Diet—A Doctor's Plan to Eliminate Hunger,
Change Your Body Chemistry, Lose Weight, and Keep
It Off.*
Luis A. Guerra, M.D. Crown Publishers, New York,
1982.

Activate the body's own appetite suppressants, stim-
ulants, and substances that burn fat. Meat, vegetables, no sweets, and the speed and sequence of eating
are important.

Fat Destroyer Foods — The Magic Metabolizer Diet.
Sidney Petrie. Parker Publishing, West Nyack NY,
1974.

End the carbohydrate conspiracy and start the protein
revolution, by paying attention to "carbo-cals."

The Hilton Head Metabolism Diet.
Dr. Peter Miller. Warner Books, New York, 1983.

Teach your body to burn off more fat by overcoming
metabolic suppression, including 20 minutes of "fun"
exercise.

Mary Ellen's Help Yourself Diet Plan.
Mary Ellen Pinkham. St. Martin's, New York, 1983.

Understand and utilize the principles of thermogenesis to control your metabolism. A low-fat diet, five walks a week, and as we would expect from the Queen of Hints, lots of helpful ones.

Chemical and Other Body Changes

The Beverly Hills Diet—How to Be as Thin as You Like for the Rest of Your Life.
Judy Mazel. Macmillan, New York, 1981.

Promote enzyme action by conscious combining of foods in your stomach so you eventually can eat all you want of anything but diet soda and artificial sweeteners. First week: mostly pineapples and papayas. Eleventh day: nothing but 3½ bagels and 3 buttered ears of corn.

The Body Clock Diet—The Newest Way to Fast and Permanent Weight Loss.
Ronald Gatty. Simon & Schuster, New York, 1978.

When you eat is far more important than what. Calories are treated differently at different times of the day. Learn your body rhythms and eat at the right time for you.

California Weight Loss Program (to Master Food Control).
H. S. Judd. Simon & Schuster, New York, 1974.

Nine intensive days to learn portion control and proper eating behavior.

Diet for Health.
Maxine Bush and Edward Fewer. Bush & Fewer, Mehoopany PA, 1951.

The proper balance of water, chlorophyll, fats and oils; no condiments, spices, or canned foods.

Dr. Cooper's Fabulous Fructose Diet.
J. T. Cooper, M.D. M. Evans, New York, 1979.

Most dieters can't handle glucose, which prevents weight loss. Eat pure fructose, fructose-laden foods, and lots of liquid.

Dr. Jolliffe's Reduce and Stay Reduced.
Norman Jolliffe, M.D. Simon & Schuster, New York, 1957.

The only vital thing is to learn to regulate your Appestat, the automatic weight-reducing "mechanism" at the base of the skull.

Dr. Romano's Megatetics Weight Reduction Guide.
Ronald Romano, D.C. Parker Publishing, West Nyack NY, 1978.

Claim is up to 25 pounds a week, 50 a month, using Tums or other heartburn pills to reduce absorption of food into the digestive tract.

Doctor's Amazing Speed Reducing Diet.
Rex Adams. Parker Publishing, West Nyack NY, 1979.

Foods with "reverse calories" — the more you eat, the more you lose. Neutralize fattening foods, too. Includes many fruits and vegetables, buffalo, clams, turtles, oysters, lobster.

The Easy No-FLAB Diet—A Safe, Reliable Nutritionist-Approved Diet That Reduces Flab along with Weight.
Richard Passwater. Richard Maret Publishers, New York, 1979.

Count FLAB (fat-liquidating-ability barometer) units, which help burn fat and preserve lean tissue.

Eat, Drink, and Get Thin.
Ernst R. Reinsh, M.D. Hart Publishing, New York,
1969.

Obesity is not fat, it is waterlogged starch. Eliminate
by avoiding apples, soft drinks (including diet ones),
flour. All meats, however fatty, are permitted.

*A Matter of Taste — Doctor's Discovery for Permanent
Weight Control.*
John Pisacano, M.D. Frederick Fell Publishers, New
York, 1979.

The key is taste control. Anaesthetize the tongue
with benzocaine chewing gum and lose the desire to
eat.

*The New Enzyme Catalyst Diet — Amazing Way to
Quick Permanent Weight Loss.*
Carlson Wede. Parker Publishing, West Nyack NY,
1976.

Fruits, vegetables to short-circuit appetite for high-
calorie foods and eliminate fat-creating oxygen buildup
in cells.

Oriental 7-Day Quick Weight-Off Diet.
Norvell (advisor to the beautiful people). Parker Publishing, West Nyack NY, 1975.

Uses foods which are claimed to take more calories
to digest than they supply, so the more the better,
including cabbage, tomatoes, celery, and lots of
brown rice.

Pounds and Inches — A New Approach to Obesity.
Simeons Medical Supply, Los Angeles.

Obesity is an abnormal kind of fat which diets can't
remove. HCG, a growth hormone from the urine of
pregnant women, plus a 500-calorie-a-day diet works.

Shape Up America — A Diet for the New Era.
Ceil Dyer. G. P. Putnam's Sons, New York, 1978.

Combinations of food can trigger a weight and water loss when neither food alone would. No sugar, lots of liquids, small portions, and no second helpings.

The Slendernow Diet — A Nutritionally Sound Program Using Two Protein Milkshakes and a Full Meal Each Day.
Richard Passwater. St. Martin's Press, New York, 1982.

An eight-week regimen of the shakes and a well-balanced third meal.

The Yogatronic Diet — Amazing New Way to a Youthful Trim Body.
Frank Young, D.C. Parker Publishing, West Nyack NY, 1979.

Absorbing the "odic force" given off by all foods, maintaining alkaline balance, and a balanced diet, keeps you slim and healthy. Visualizing the food as you eat it.

Inspiration

The Beautiful People's Diet Book.
Luciana Avedon. E. P. Dutton, New York, 1973.

Heat lamps, massage, towel flagellation, a low-calorie diet, and the sincere desire to be a beautiful person.

Build a Better and Slimmer You.
Jean Allen. Arlington House, New Rochelle NY, 1977.

Obesity clinic narrative on how she was retrained and educated to a life of counting calories and eating fewer of them.

Dr. Rader's No Diet Program for Permanent Weight Loss.
William Rader, M.D. J. P. Tarcher, Los Angeles, 1979.

Techniques learned in working with Alcoholics Anonymous. Working with a diet partner to talk to in times of stress. Learn *why* you eat, not what, when, or how.

Doctor Schiff's Miracle Weight Loss Guide — A Fresh, Comprehensive, and Different Approach to the Problems of Overweight and Obesity.
Martin Schiff, M.D. Parker Publishing, West Nyack NY, 1974.

Food for thought is the most important food, along with a high-protein, low-fat, low-carbohydrate diet.

The Fat Is in Your Head.
Reverend Charlie Shedd. Word Publishing, 1972.

A combination of prayer, behavior modification, and evangelism.

Free to Be Thin.
Marie Chapian. Bethany Fellowship, Minneapolis, 1979.

Find God and get thin. Eat Kingdom Foods: low fat, natural food, not World Food (desserts, artificial sweeteners); plus prayer.

The Greatest Diet in the World.
Dolly Dimples. Chateau Publishing, Orlando FL, 1968.

The famous circus fat lady lost 443 pounds through faith in God, no salt, and 800 calories a day.

How the Doctors Diet.
Peter and Barbara Wyden. Trident Press, New York, 1968.

Interviews with 89 physicians, including some famous diet doctors, to learn what they do (or, in many cases, don't do but wish they had time to do).

The Meditation Diet — The Relaxation System for Easy Weight Loss.
Richard Tyson, M.D. Playboy Press, Chicago, 1976.

Reducing tension reduces appetite. Learn meditation to reduce tension and eat less.

The Partnership Diet Program.
Kelly Brownell. Rawson, Wade Publishers, New York, 1980.

Write everything down and discuss with your weight-loss partner (mate, friend, etc.). 800 to 1,200 calories a day, but no set meal plan.

The Psychologist's Eat-Anything Diet — The Scientific New System of Permanent Pleasurable Weight Control for Liberated Eating.
Dr. Leonard Pearson. Peter Wyden, New York, 1973.

Increased awareness of body and desires in relation to foods that "hum and beckon." The body will learn to regulate itself.

Regimen for Weight Control.
Charles Aronson. CNA Book Publisher, Arcade NY, 1973.

Eat anything you want in any quantity once you have learned to eat only two meals a day.

Weight Control Through Yoga.
Richard Hittleman. Bantam Books, New York, 1971.

Mind over matter, meditation, and besides, the thinner you get, the more advanced yoga positions you will be able to do.

You Can Do It.
William Proxmire. Simon & Schuster, New York, 1973.

How the Senator keeps trim with a large breakfast, fruit for lunch, and nothing but a single portion of meat or fish for dinner.

Biofeedback and Lollipops

The Biofeedback Diet—A Doctor's Revolutionary Approach.
J. Frank Hurdle, M.D. Parker Publishing, West Nyack NY, 1977.

Stop depression, set your biological clock, gain control of your metabolism, control headache, and control the vagus nerves that start gastric juices flowing, by learning biofeedback techniques.

A Sweet Way to Diet.
Sonja Eiteljorg. Doubleday, New York, 1968.

A balanced diet plus three lollipops a day, because they satisfy the sweet tooth while taking so long and so much energy to eat.

Non-Gimmick Low-Calorie Balanced Diets

The Bronx Diet.
Richard Smith. Workman Publishing, New York, 1979.

An amusing book offering this "radical principle": to reduce, eat less.

Diet for Life—The New Joyous Way to Permanent Slimness, High Energy, Sexual Vigor, Glowing Physical and Mental Health, and Added Youthful Years.
Francine Prince. Simon & Schuster, New York, 1981.

Low-fat, low-cholesterol, no sugar, no salt gourmet diet, with modest exercise.

A Diet for Living.
Jean Mayer. David McKay, New York, 1975.

No fads, fakes, or fallacies. Nothing dramatic or controversial. Just practical advice.

The Easy 24-Hour Diet.
Marvin Small. Doubleday, Garden City NY, 1973.

This means to take it one day at a time. Emphasis on keeping portion sizes large, but with reduced-calorie ingredients (such as mixing lots of watercress in with the ground beef).

Eat Yourself Slim.
Shirley Bright Boody. Gramercy Publishing, New York, 1968.

Three meals and three snacks a day, totalling less food, but all carefully balanced.

How to Gorge George Without Feeding Fanny.
Nancy Gould. Hawthorn Books, New York, 1970.

The good-food-craving author, a model, lost 44 pounds with her own gourmet low-calorie well-balanced recipes, created to make or match her moods.

Ladies' Home Journal Family Diet Book.
Frances Evans. Macmillan, New York, 1973.

1,200 calories a day, based on choosing specific units from six basic food groups (milk, protein, fruit, vegetables, breads, fats).

The Prudent Diet.
Iva Bennett. Bantam Books, New York, 1974.

Balanced low-calorie, low-saturated-fats, low-cholesterol meal plan.

The San Francisco Weight Loss Method — The Proven Way to Permanent Thin.
David Schoenstadt, M.D. E. P. Dutton, New York, 1975.

Overall health program, eliminating "bogeyman" foods, and exchanging foods with equal caloric, fat, carbohydrate, and protein content from lists of recommended foods.

Think and Grow Thin — Your New Way of Life Method for Keeping Slender.
Joan and Dr. Morton Walker. Arco Publishing,
New York, 1973.

The New York City Obesity Clinic's plan for physiological bookkeeping. Count calories, low fat, high
vegetable, no sweets.

Winning the Diet Wars — A Rescue Plan for Those Who Love to Eat.
Meridee Merzer. Harcourt Brace Jovanovich,
New York, 1980.

Light but scholarly look at dieting, with a Sensible
1200 Diet, evolved from the same New York City
Health Department diet that was the basis for the
Weight Watchers diet.

On paper, it makes a terrific amount of sense. Just as the tiny drops of water collect to form a mighty river, so do the tiniest drops in caloric intake during normal eating behavior collect into mighty rivers of fat, streaming away forever. As it were.

If your weight is stable now (even if you are greatly overweight), and if you do *nothing* but leave out one little pat of butter a day, you will lose almost 1/10th of a pound a week. This tiny drop doesn't sound like a big deal, but it turns into a loss of 50 pounds over the next 10 years.

The following chart lists a bunch of things that are commonly eaten, and which probably wouldn't be missed a whole lot if they *weren't* eaten occasionally. By eliminating *all* the portions listed in the chart, and changing nothing else, your weight presumably would drop by 81 pounds per year, for a total of 810 pounds over the next ten years.

Since this is hardly necessary for most of us, the other way of looking at it is that if you only do *2 to 10 percent* of these things, and all else remains unchanged, you will still lose significant amounts of weight, albeit rather slowly. *Or* you can do everything on this list (or equivalents) and should decline by upwards of 80 pounds a year.

The reason I say, a bit wistfully, that this splendid philosophy probably won't work for me, is that my eating habits are not that regular, nor do I especially want them to be. I can go for weeks or months without putting butter on bread, but then I'll rediscover that pleasure and slather it on thickly for a while. That sort of thing.

Still, it sure does make a lot of sense. I may reconsider. Any day now. Yes.

If you reduce your intake of this substance...	by this much ...	then in ten years, you'll be this much lighter
Bacon	3 strips twice a week	50 pounds
Beer	2 cans a week	50 pounds
Biscuits	2 a week	50 pounds
Bread	1 slice a day	60 pounds
Butter	1 pat a day	50 pounds
Candy bar (small)	1 per week	30 pounds
Cheese	2 ounces a week	30 pounds
Cookie (medium)	1 a day	60 pounds
Cream	1 teaspoon a day	20 pounds
Doughnut	2 a week	40 pounds
Eggs, scrambled	2 eggs a week	30 pounds
French fries	1 serving a week	30 pounds
Ham	1 medium slice a week	50 pounds
Ice cream	1 scoop a week	20 pounds
Mayonnaise	4 tablespoons a week	40 pounds
Pizza	2 slices a week	30 pounds
Potato chips	20 chips a week	30 pounds
Rice	1 cup a week	20 pounds
Soda	4 cans a week	60 pounds
Sugar	2 teaspoons a day	40 pounds
Wine	2 glasses a week	20 pounds

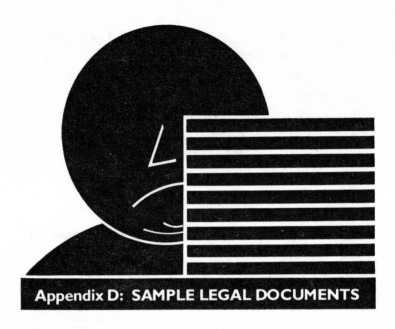

Sample Trust Agreement for Weight Loss

This Trust Agreement, made and entered into this _____ day of _____ in the year 19_____, by and between (*your name, your address*), hereinafter referred to as Grantor, and (*name of your trustee, address of your trustee*), hereinafter referred to as Trustee.

Whereas the Grantor presently weighs (*current weight*) pounds, as determined by (*method of determining,* such as "weighing by Dr. John Smith, with offices at *address*"), by a weight measurement on the scale of (*person doing weighing*), in the ordinary and usual manner of measuring the weight of patients for physical examinations (*if weigher is a doctor*), and

Whereas the Grantor is desirous of weighing _____ pounds or less on or before (*goal date*), and

Whereas, in order to lose said weight, Grantor believes that a monetary incentive is better for him than a medical or cosmetic incentive, and

Whereas the Grantor believes that (*name of pledge recipient,* for instance "the American Nazi Party [also known as the National Socialist White People's Party] of Arlington, Virginia") is one of the most despicable, undesirable, and dangerous organizations in the United States today,

Now Therefore, in consideration of the Trust hereby assumed by the said Trustee, and of the mutual covenants contained herein, it is agreed as follows:

1. The Grantor hereby deposits with the Trustee the sum of (*amount of pledge*) which the Trustee will deposit in his own escrow account in (*name of bank, number of account*).

2. On or before (*goal date*), Grantor will appear at the office of (*name of physician or other weigher*) or of any other physician of his own choosing, in order to be weighed in the same manner as set out above. Grantor shall then instruct the said physician to certify in writing to the Trustee the results of said weighing.

3. In the event that the weight of the Grantor, as certified by said physician, shall exceed (*goal weight*) pounds, or in the event Grantor shall fail to be so weighed on or before (*goal date*), for any reason whatsoever, other than the physical incapacity of the Grantor, or for reasons beyond his control, the Trustee shall immediately set over and transfer said (*amount of pledge*), plus any accumulated interest, to the (*recipient of pledge*) by certified or registered mail.

4. If the designated recipient is unwilling to accept the amount of the Trust, or cannot be located, then said Trust shall be transferred in the same manner to (*alternative recipient, address*).

5. In the event that the weight, as certified by said physician, is (*goal weight*) or less, or in the event Grantor shall not be so weighed on or before (*goal date*) for reasons of physical incapacity, or for reasons beyond his control, the Trustee shall return said pledge amount to Grantor, and this Trust shall be considered fully terminated.

6. The Trustee shall have the sole discretion to determine if the Grantor was prevented from being weighed as required above for reasons beyond the control of said Grantor.

7. The Trustee acting hereunder shall not be required to furnish any bond or security for the performance of his duties hereunder.

8. Upon the death of the Trustee hereunder, (*alternative name and address*) shall act as Successor Trustee hereunder.

9. The Trustee, by joining in the execution hereof, acknowledges receipt of the said Trust, and signifies acceptance of the Trust hereby granted.

In Witness Whereof, the Grantor and Trustee have hereunto set their respective hands and seals the day and year first above written.

———————————————————————

(*Your Name*), Grantor

———————————————————————

(*Trustee's Name*), Trustee

Sample Trust Agreement for
Weight Maintenance

This Trust Agreement, made and entered into this
_____ day of _____, 19_____, by and
between (*your name*) of (*address*), hereinafter
referred to as Grantor, and (*trustee's name*) of
(*trustee's address*), hereinafter referred to as Trustee.

Whereas the Grantor is desirous of maintaining his
weight at (*goal weight*), or less, and

Whereas, in order not to exceed said weight, Grantor
believes a monetary incentive is better for him than a
medical or cosmetic incentive, and

Whereas Grantor believes that (*potential recipient of
pledge*) of (*address*) is one of the most despicable,
undesirable, and dangerous organizations in the
United States today,

Now Therefore, in consideration of the Trust hereby
assumed by said Trustee, and of the mutual covenants
contained herein, it is agreed as follows:

1. The Grantor hereby deposits with the Trustee
   (*amount of pledge*). The Grantor reserves the right
   to substitute cash, negotiable securities, precious
   metals, or other objects with a clear cash value at
   any time, as long as the substitution is equal to or
   greater in value than the deposit.

2. On or before (*weigh-in date*), and every six (6)
   months thereafter, Grantor will appear at the
   office of (*name of physician or other, address*), or at
   the office of any other licensed physician of his own
   choosing, in order to be weighed in the ordinary
   and usual manner of measuring the weight of
   patients for physical examinations, after which
   Grantor shall then instruct said physician to certify
   in writing to the Trustee the results of said
   weighing.

3. In the event the weight of Grantor as certified by said physician shall exceed (*goal weight*), the Trustee shall immediately pay to (*recipient number one*), or, if said party shall no longer be in existence, to (*alternative recipient*), a sum equal to (*amount of money,* for instance $100) per pound for each pound over (*goal weight*).

4. In the event the Grantor shall fail to be so weighed on any weighing-in date for any reason whatsoever, other than the physical incapacity of the Grantor, or for reasons beyond his control, Trustee shall immediately set over and transfer the entire amount of the Trust to (*recipient number one*), or, in the event said party is no longer in existence, to (*alternative recipient*).

5. This Agreement shall continue through the weighing-in date of (*date in future,* suggested to be at least 5 years away), and thereafter for periods as set out by written direction of the Grantor.

6. At the termination of this Agreement, or at the termination of any extended period of this Agreement, the Trustee shall return the amount or content of the Trust in his possession to the Grantor, provided Grantor has maintained his weight at (*goal weight*) or less, and has complied with all the provisions of this Agreement.

7. The Trustee shall have the sole discretion to determine if the Grantor was prevented from being weighed as required above for reasons beyond the control of the said Grantor.

8. Any income, or dividends, or stock dividends which may become payable on any security in the possession of said Trustee during the term of or any extended term of this Agreement, shall be the property of the Grantor.

9. The Trustee acting hereunder shall not be required to furnish any bond or security for the performance of his duties hereunder.

10. Upon the death of the Trustee hereunder, (*alternative trustee, address*) shall act as Successor Trustee hereunder.

11. The Trustee, by joining in the execution hereof, acknowledges receipt of the said Trust, and signifies acceptance of the Trust hereby granted.

In Witness Whereof, the Grantor and Trustee have hereunto set their respective hands and seals the day and year first above written.

_____

(*Your Name*), Grantor

_____

(*Trustee's Name*), Trustee